NEW MEDICAL FRONTIERS, INC.

>>><<<

I0767247

BOOK
OF
NATURAL HEALTH
Your Source of Health & Longevity

Volume 5

50 chapters, scientifically validated

Dr. Mark Fritz, NMD, PhD

>>><<<

Copyright © Dr. Mark Fritz, New Medical Frontiers, Inc. 2024

ISBN: 9798883781505

All rights reserved.
No part of this publication may be reproduced, stored in a retrieval system, or transmitted, in any form or by any means, electronic, mechanical, photocopying, recording, or otherwise, without the written prior permission of the author.

DISCLAIMER

The content of this book is for informational purposes only and is not intended to replace the advice and treatment by a healthcare provider. Every metabolism is different. Work with your physician/healthcare provider to find the best solutions for your heath.

All contents of this book are commentary or opinion and are protected under Free Speech Laws in all civilized countries. The information is provided for educational and entertainment purposes only and is not intended to diagnose, treat, cure, or prevent any condition or disease. Dr. Mark Fritz assumes no responsibility for the use or misuse of this material. No warranty of any kind, whether expressed or implied, is given in relation to this information or any of the external services referred to. This is a comprehensive limitation of liability that applies to all damages of any kind, including (without limitation) compensatory, direct, indirect or consequential damages.

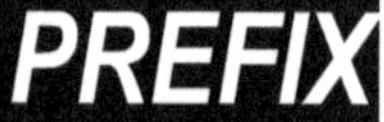

This is the 5th volume of the series "Books of Natural Health" for citizens and patients, who understand that they themselves are primarily responsible for their most precious good in life – their health – which, to be sure, is based on laws of nature.

Doing justice accordingly, 2 avenues to make use of this book best:

- Read it from chapter 1-50 for your information/education.
- You find hundreds of health issues covered with at least one recommended natural solution each. With appropriate natural remedies and modalities, as indicated alphabetically in "index".

See exact scientific validations by almost 350 U.S. and international universities/medical schools and research institutions – all listed in alphabetical order at the end in 'references'.

Dr. Mark Fritz, NMD, PhD
President
of
New Medical Frontiers, Inc.

a leading independent documentation & information center for latest scientific breakthroughs in natural/naturopathic medicine on a global basis

www.newmedicalfrontiers.com

CONTENTS

Instead of an own

FOREWORD

"An ounce of prevention is worth a pound of cure."

Benjamin Franklin
(1706-1790)
Scientist
&
Founding Father of the United States

1. EXOTIC FRUIT FOR YOUR HEALTH

THE PHILOSOPHY BEHIND

As you know from our latest publications, healthy diet – besides physical .exercise – is one of the 2 basic pillars for our health and longevity. With special reference to fruits. Dependent on their natural content of certain vitamins, minerals, antioxidants, and other specific nutrients. While the knowledge about our native fruits – regardless where you live – has been passed on from generation to generation, there are well some fruits entering our culture from abroad. Although these are not necessarily disadvantageous for our health and longevity, it is still important to know about their nutritious background. To understand where exactly the benefits are. In this respect, we picked 3 exotic fruits for you, as follows.

LYCHEE/PERSIMMON/STAR FRUITS – SCIENTIFICALLY VERIFIED

Lychees

Basically native to tropical and sub-tropical China and India, and historically known and used there already 2000 B.C., this fruit comes from the evergreen tree *litchi chinensis*. Conventionally named *lychee*, it is also going by the botanical names
- Chinese cherry
- lychee nut
  &
- litchi

Especially loaded with *vitamin C* and *antioxidants*, this fruit has benefits for our health in terms of being
- anti-diabetic
- anti-carcinogenic
- anti-inflammatory
- cardioprotective
  &
- anti-angiogenic
  (preventing tumors from growing new blood vessels)

According to research at, inter alia,
- *South China Agricultural University* in Guangzhou
  &
- *Zhejiang University* in Hangzhou

(both China)
- *Kobe University* in Kobe, Japan
  &
- *University of Palermo* in Palermo, Italy

Based on research at *Andhra University* in Andhra Pradesh, India, lychee fruits may
- inhibit cancer cells & viruses
  &
- protect the liver

Persimmon

In fact, there are 2 types of persimmon fruits.

One of the 2 types of persimmon fruit - *diospyros virginiana* – has been known by the native Americans already 300 years ago.

The other type - *diospyros kaki* – is native to Japan, ripening there between September and December.

Split up in 2 subtypes:

The acorn-shaped *hachiya* and the tomato-shaped *fuyu* - both comparable in terms of health benefits.

With special reference to vitamin A giving *persimmons* the power to support
- eye health & vision.

Based on research at, inter alia, the *University of Washington* in Seattle, WA.

Another benefit is the high load of antioxidants to help with, inter alia,
- cancer
- diabetes
- cardiovascular disease
  &
- Alzheimer's disease

according to research at, inter alia, *Stanford University Medical Center* in Palo Alto, CA.

Not to overlook the anti-inflammatory power of this fruit due to its high content of vitamin C helping, inter alia, with
-    heart disease
based on research at, inter alia, the *University of Connecticut* Storrs, CT,
-    prostate cancer
according to research at *Dalian University of Technology* in Dalian, China
&
-    diabetes
according to research at, inter alia, *Harbin Medical University* in Harbin, China

Also to mention *persimmon*'s high content of fiber helping to
-    remove high cholesterol
from the body.

As based on research at the *University* of *Nebraska-Lincoln* in lincoln, NE and *Clemson University* in Clemson, SC.

Star Fruit

This is another exotic (star shaped) fruit from Southeast Asia, also named 'carambola' ('cane apple') in its original Malayan language.

Loaded with powerful nutrients such as, inter alia,
-    vitamin C
     &
-    minerals like magnesium, calcium and potassium
according to the *U.S. Department of Agriculture*.

Especially important, as vitamin C produces *collagen* as a substance the self-healing power of our body is dependent on.

Along with star fruit's impressive content of fiber to reduce high cholesterol and the risk of cardiovascular disease.

In fact, according to its native Ayurvedic & traditional Chinese medicine, star fruit has been used since many centuries to treat, inter alia,
-    fever
-    headache
-    cough
-    sore throat
-    asthma
     &
-    skin problems

Scientifically verified today with special reference to, inter alia,
- cardiovascular disease
  (*University of Colombo* in Colombo, Sri Lanka)
  &
- reducing high cholesterol from the body
- (*City University of New York* in New York City, NY)

IN A NUTSHELL

Since mankind is on this planet, the earth, for millions of years, its health was – and still is – supported by nature's healthy food with its powerful nutrients. Globally, including those exotic fruits you learned about in this outline. Scientifically verified internationally today.

2. WESTERN DIET – YOUR TICKET TO DEATH?

THE PHILOSOPHY BEHIND

As you have learned from our publications and seminars, support of our health & longevity depends on 2 basic pillars: physical activity and healthy diet. With special reference to health of our heart.

Healthy diet? Being proud of our Western heritage and culture most of us, we may believe that healthy diet is automatically part of it. Called *Western diet*. Unfortunately yet, there is a myth behind.

In fact, despite of spending highest amount for medicine per capita, unhealthy food is responsible for almost half of cardiovascular deaths in the U.S. According to the U.S. *National Institute of Health (NIH)* in Bethesda, MD.

Even more, heart failure is the #1 of unsolved health problems in the Western world, leading to premature death, followed by cancer and diabetes.

SCIENTIFIC SCRUTINY OF WESTERN DIET

Based on the fact that our seemingly progressive (?) Western diet is loaded with saturated fat, trans fat, sodium and cholesterol. Leading to the front yard of heart disease such as *atherosclerosis*, i.e. a related disorder influencing elasticity of arteries negatively by buildup of fatty plaques on artery walls, narrowing blood vessels, accordingly. With heart failure as a potential consequence.

- *Fats*

High-fat diet as part of the Western diet has a negative impact also on white blood cells which are the first line of defense against infections. Even a single high-fat meal can have a negative effect on blood vessels, based on research at *Augusta University* and the *Medical College of Georgia* in Augusta, GA.

Especially 2 types of fats are debilitating and potentially causing heart attack:
- saturated fats (mainly in meat and dairy) and

- trans fats (mainly in commercially baked foods, certain margarines, solid cooking fats and deep-fried food prepared with hardened vegetable oils)

Scientifically verified also by
- *Harvard T.H. Chan School of Public Health*
- *Harvard Medical School*
  and
- *Brigham and Women's Hospital* in Boston, MA
  as well as
- *Cleveland Clinic* in Lyndhurst, Ohio.

Even worse, according to research at, inter alia, the
- *University of Iowa* in Iowa City, Iowa
  &
- *Washington University School of Medicine* in St. Louis, MO
especially females aged over 50 are enhancing their premature cardiovascular death risk by regular consumption of fried foods.

Such as, inter alia,
- fried chicken
- fried fish, shellfish (like shrimp or oysters), and fish sandwich,
- French fries, tortilla chips, tacos, etc.

This is in line with the results of a meta-analysis developed, inter alia, in China at

- *Shenzhen University School of Medicine* in Schenzhen
- *Zhengzhou University* in Zhengzhou
- *University of Chinese Academy of Sciences Shenzhen Hospital* in Shenzhen

according to which the consumption of fried foods may well be linked not only to cardiovascular events but also enhance the level of 'bad' (LDL) cholesterol, lowering 'good' (HDL) cholesterol at the same time.

- ### *Sodium*

Just as too much salt (sodium) in this type of Western diet may raise blood pressure, as another related cardiovascular disorder.

While, according to the *American Heart Association (AHA)*, salt intake should be limited to 1,500 milligrams (mg) up to 2,300 mg highest per day, average consumption in the U.S. is more than 3,400 mg per capita and day.

- ***Other***

Also, a shortage of fruits and vegetables in our diet, thus lacking life-supporting vitamins, minerals (such as potassium and magnesium), fiber, and antioxidants, is a potential key to heart-related deaths.

According to research at, inter alia,
- *Harvard School of Public Health*
  &
- *Tufts University*
  both in Boston, US-State of Massachusetts
  as well as
- *Huazhong University of Science and Technology* in Wuhan, China.

Another counterproductive nutritional factor with respect to heart health is protein-rich meat. While this type of protein-rich food is considered beneficial for weight loss and muscle-buildup, it may well be counterproductive for the cardiovascular system because of their content of sulfur amino acids. Primarily *methionine* as an essential amino acid, *cysteine,* as a semi-essential amino acid. At least if they are consumed in high quantities.

These findings are especially relevant as, according to research at *Washington University School of Medicine* in St. Louis, MO, this type of protein-rich food is not only unfavorable for cardiovascular health but may increase heart attack risk specifically.

Therefore, according to research at, inter alia,
- *Harvard T.H. Chan School of Public Health* in Boston, MA,
- *Pennsylvania State University* in University Park, PA,
- *Louisiana State University System* in Baton Rouge, LA, *and*
- *Universita Vita-Salute San Raffaele* in Milan, Italy,

red meat should be replaced with plant protein sources. with heart-healthy benefit.

WAY OUT

In fact, not all cultures in our Western hemisphere are alike. Nutrition being no exception.

Just take the statistics on life expectancy of the *World Health Organization*. While countries north and south of the *Mediterranean Sea* (that part of the Earth where *Man* was created 2 and a half million years ago) are on top of the scale, the U.S. is trailing behind at position 31. Let's take a closer look at the *Mediterranean diet* as a feasible alternative.

According to research at, inter alia,
- *Harvard Medical School*
- *Harvard T.H. Chan School of Public Health* and
- *Brigham and Women's Hospital* all in Boston, MA as well as the Canadian
- *Population Health Research Institute (PHRI)* in Hamilton/Ontario

Mediterranean diet – rich in plants and olive oil but low in meat and sugary products - reduces the risk of cardiovascular disease by a quarter, with special reference to coronary heart disease, stroke and heart attack.

Scientifically verified also by the *Center for Genetics, Nutrition, and Health* in Washington, D.C.

Although there are some varieties of Mediterranean diet, all rely on the same basic nutrients, as recommended and validated, inter alia, by the *American Heart Association*. Such as, inter alia,
- high volume of vegetables and fruits
- nuts and seeds
- high fiber starches like beans, potatoes, whole grain bread, etc.
- poultry and fish
- eggs up to 4 times a week &
- whole grain

Only recently, *Tufts University* in Boston, MA, has concluded scientifically that consuming more whole grain reduces the risk of cardiovascular disease.

Another important part of Mediterranean diet is

- olive oil

    which not only controls blood pressure, but also reduces risk of atrial fibrillation (A-fib).

According to a Spanish mega-study based on research at
- *University of Barcelona* in Barcelona
- *University of Las Palmas de Gran Canaria* in Las Palmas
- *University of Malaga* in Malaga
- *University of Valencia* in Valencia
- *University of Navarra* in Pamplona
- *Hospital Universitari de Sant Joan de Reus*

Also, mono-unsaturated fats in olive oil are controlling weight.
(Please note: mono- and poly-unsaturated oils from olives, soybeans, canola and corn are free of trans fats.)

In fact, the U.S. *Food and Drug Administration* has agreed that olive oil is heart healthy with its monounsaturated fat which cuts down the risk of coronary heart disease. Keeping arteries unblocked to support unhampered flow of blood with oxygen and nutrients to the heart.

At the same time Mediterranean diet is low in
- (especially red) meat
- dairy-fat
- junk food

Scientifically verified also by the *Universities of East Anglia, Cambridge* and *Aberdeen* in the UK, and *McMaster University* in Hamilton/Ontario, Canada.

According to this research, Mediterranean diet may reduce the risk of stroke by 17%. Especially for women aged 40 years plus.

IN A NUTSHELL

If you favor our Western culture, its so called *Western diet* may still harm your health, and heart specifically. Unless you adjust your nutritional pattern naturally in favor of your health and longevity.

3. WHAT IS HEALTHY DIET ALL ABOUT?

THE PHILOSOPHY BEHIND

We certainly love tasty food saturating us. Whatever it is, as long as we like it. However, yes, there is a 'philosophy behind' many of us tend to overlook: nutrition is basically important to support our body and mind for health and longevity. Along with physical exercise. As the center core our complex and comprehensive biologic-ecologic existence is built on.

If we ignore this fact, chances are to develop highly debilitating illnesses like those listed on the *World Health Organization* statistics of 'chronic' diseases with heart failure on top. And also to become overweight/obese later in life.

Leaves us with the question which nutrients are important to make our foods really healthy – and which are counterproductive? Starting in fact in the womb with diet during pregnancy, and breastfeeding.

Let's ask the most competent institution for health on this globe:

DIETARY GUIDELINES OF THE WORLD HEALTH ORGANIZATION

Although gender, age, pattern physical activity and other lifestyle factors play a role in our life, there are still basics in our nutrition to observe, as follows according to the *World Health Organization (WHO)* for our population. Young and old alike.

Scientifically verified also, inter alia, by the *Harvard Schol of Public Health* in Boston, MA.

Adults

- Plant-based diet:
  Consume at least 400 g of total fruits/vegetables/nuts/whole grains/legumes (lentils/beans) per day.
  Excluding regular & sweet potatoes, cassava & other starchy foods.
  Thereby, the intake of fruits & vegetables may be improved by, inter alia,
    - including vegetables in meals regularly
    - consuming fruits & vegetables in season

- prefer a whole variety of fruits & vegetables
- eat raw vegetables & fresh fruits as snacks

- Fats:
  Cut down on
  - saturated fats as found in fatty meat/palm & coconut oil/butter/cream/cheese/ghee/lard
    as well as on
  - trans fats as prevalent in baked/fried foods and pre-packed snacks and foods like frozen pizzas/cookies/pies/wafers/biscuits/cooking oils & spreads as well as dairy foods from ruminant animals like cows/goats/sheep/camels

  Thereby, intake of saturated and trans fats can be reduced by
  - replacing frying by steaming/boiling
  - replacing butter/ghee/lard by polyunsaturated fats like soybean/canola (rapeseed)/sunflower/corn/safflower oils
  - eating lean meats

Consume unsaturated fats like in fish/nuts/avocados as well as soybean/canola/olive oils.

- Sugars:
  Especially cut down on free sugars as added to foods/drinks by manufacturer or as being present in syrups/fruit juices/fruit juice concentrates.

  To manage not only weight control and the risk of dental caries but also cardiovascular disease.

  Reduce sugar intake by limiting
  - sugary snacks
  - candies
  - sugar-sweetened beverages like fruit/vegetable juices
  - sports drinks
  - ready-to-drink-tea/coffee
  - flavored milk drinks

- Salt:
  Restrict sodium to less than one teaspoon per day.

This is especially important as high sodium/low potassium intake may lead to high blood pressure with the potential heart disease & stroke.

In fact, most sodium comes from processed foods like
- ready meals
- processed meats (like bacon/salami/ham)
- salty snacks
- cheese

To lower salt intake, limit consumption of salty snacks & high sodium sauces as well as high sodium condiments (such as fish sauce/soy sauce/bouillon)

Infants & young children

Although basically, this population group may be fed like adults, but with slight adjustments such as, inter alia,
- Breastfeeding exclusively only first 6 months of life
- From 6 months on, complement breastmilk with adequate/safe/nutrient-dense foods
- Don't add salt/sugar to complementary foods

IN A NUTSHELL

In order to reduce the risk of highly debilitating disease (like, inter alia, heart failure, cancer, diabetes) and premature death, healthy diet, besides physical activity, plays the central role. In this chapter you learned about those nutritional criteria to look at in favor of your health and life expectancy.

4. HOW AVERT DIABETES NATURALLY?

THE PHILOSOPHY BEHIND

Despite of progressive conventional medicine, diabetes is one of the most debilitating diseases in our industrialized society. Even more, according to the World Health Organization (WHO), it is in the top region of so called 'chronic' diseases with manifold premature death.

Not enough, the most prescribed medication for diabetes worldwide, according to its producer, a major international pharmaceutical company, offers no cure but comes with more than 80 side effects. Leading, inter alia, to heart disease, stroke, kidney failure and blindness.

LIFESTYLE ADJUSTMENTS – SCIENTIFICALLY VERIFIED

Fortunately, there are life adjustments to get out of this vicious cycle naturally – powerful and without side effects.

Healthy diet

is one of those.

According to the U.S. *Centers for Disease Control and Prevention (CDC)* with special reference to

- ***Fruits***

- ***Non-starchy vegetables***
  such as
    - spinach
    - broccoli
    - mushrooms
    - asparagus

- ***Whole grains***
  like
  - steel-cut oatmeal
  - quinoa
  - brown rice

- ***Lean proteins***
  such as
  - turkey
  - fish
  - pulses
  - eggs
  - plain Greek yogurt
  - tofu
  - water
  - unsweetened beverages

At the same time

- **refrain from**

  - *sugary drinks* (like soda/fruit juice/sports drinks)
  - *trans fats* (as we find in packaged bake goods/fried foods/snack foods/margarine, etc.)
  - *processed foods* (like chips/sweets/fast foods/packaged snacks/preserved meat/granola bars)

Thereby, healthy diet helps also with

Weight management

being important to ward off diabetes.

Along with

- ***portion control***

as also recommended by the *Centers for Disease Control and Prevention (CDC)*.

To do so, fill your plate as follows:
  - one half with non-starchy vegetables
  - one-quarter with carbohydrates
  - one-quarter with protein-rich foods

Also, the American Diabetic Association (ADA) recommends following practice to lose weight naturally:

  - eat breakfast daily

- less than 10 hours of TV watching per week
- reduce consumption of fat and calories
- check your body weight once per week at same time of day to control progress
- stay active physically

Physical exercise

To help preventing diabetes, one should exercise 30 minutes daily 5 times a week.

According to the U.S. *National Institute of Diabetes and Digestive and Kidney Diseases (NIDDK).*

Control high blood pressure

According to international research at, inter alia,
- *University of Oxford* in Oxford
  &
- *University of Manchester* in Manchester
  (both UK)
  as well as
- *University of Sydney* in Sydney, Australia

high blood pressure is a risk factor of diabetes.

Therefore, the *American Diabetic Association* recommends to, inter alia,
- eating whole grain cereals
- consuming foods with less than 400 mg of sodium per serving
- replace salt by spices and herbs for flavoring

Relaxation

Stress is also a risk factor of diabetes, to be tackled with

- *Yoga*

according to research at, inter alia, the *Government Medical College* in Kozhikode, India.
Another way to support relaxation is

- *Meditation*

especially in cases of coronary artery disease, according to research in India at *Government Medical College* in Banda & *Maulana Azad Medical College* in New Delhi.

Stop smoking

According to the U.S. *Centers for Disease Control and Prevention (CDC),* the risk of smokers to attract diabetes is roughly 1/3 higher than that of non-smokers.

Therefore, the *American Diabetic Association (ADA)* recommends that smokers may do the following to stop this health wise unfavorable habit more easily.

- Set date in near future when to stop smoking definitely
- Quit smoking at same time as friends and/or family members do this as well
- Ask others for mental support
- Trash cigarettes/lighters/ashtrays

IN A NUTSHELL

Diabetes is one of most debilitating and chronic diseases in our industrialized society. Leading to equally debilitating side effects, and even premature death in many cases. Fortunately, however, it may be warded off with natural lifestyle adjustments. Like those listed in this chapter.

5. EATING RIGHT FOR LOSING WEIGHT

THE PHILOSOPHY BEHIND

Two thirds of adults in the U.S. are overweight, half of those (one third) are even obese – i.e. their weight is at least 30% higher than it should be according to their age and height.

This, however, is not only an optical issue and a matter of satiety but rather one of basic health. In terms of quantity and quality of basic nutrition.

APPROPRIATE NUTRITION – SCIENTIFICALLY VERIFIED

When we start with fruit and vegetables, we may not get the impression that primarily losing weight is primarily a matter of quantity but at same time also of quality – in terms of nutrition, in terms of a natural and balanced diet.

And doing justice accordingly, we do not have to be vegetarian or even vegan. Still, how's about fruits and vegetables in this relationship? With special reference to weight management.

- ***Fruits***

Usually, fruits are – importantly – rich in nutrients such as vitamins, minerals and fiber, and reduced in calories at the same time.

This nutritional benefit helps our health, accordingly, with special reference to manifold chronic
- Heart disease (also with high blood pressure)
  &
- Diabetes

According to research at, inter alia, *Inje University College of Medicine* in Seoul, South Korea.

Specifically avocados, rich inter alia in fiber and healthy fats, assist with weight loss management, as based on research at, inter alia, the *Avocado Nutrition Center* at Mission Viejo, CA.

When it comes to fiber, we should also know that this nutrient also slows down digestion, which is specifically important when it comes to weight loss!

- ***Vegetables***

Especially cruciferous vegetables such as
- cauliflower
- broccoli
- Brussels sprouts
  &
- cabbage

are not only high in fiber and protein but also support weight loss management.

Based on research, inter alia, in Turkey at
- *Gazi University* in the capital of Ankara
- *Cukurova University* in Adana
- &
- *Bandirama Onyedi Eylul University* in Bandirama

as well as at
- *University of Naples Federico II* in Naples, Italy

- ***Pulses***

 such as lentils/bean/peas/chickpeas, are helpful for weight management because of their fiber content for better digestion and absorption. And together with its protein they contain is giving the impression of satiety.

According to research inter alia in Florida at
- *Florida State University* Tallahassee
  &
- *University of Florida* in Gainesville

- ***Oatmeal***

With its content of protein and carbohydrates, as well as fiber, oatmeal also helps with satiety and weight loss.

Based on research inter alia at
- *University of Copenhagen* in Frederiksberg, Denmark
- *Technical University of Denmark* in Kongens Lyngby, Denmark
- *Chalmers University of Technology* in Goeteborg, Sweden
- *University of Auckland* in Auckland, New Zealand

- ***Nuts***

Similar the effect of nuts with their content of fiber/protein/heart-healthy fats for weight management.

Internationally scientifically verified at, inter alia,
- *University Medical Center Utrecht* in Utrecht, The Netherlands
- *University of Tromsoe* in Tromsoe, Norway
- *University Paris-Saclay* in Villejuif, France
- *Aarhus University* in Aarhus, Denmark
- *Imperial College London* in London, UK

- **Fish**

Rich in healthy fats and protein, specific types of fish such as
- trout
- haddock
- cod

help with weight loss.

According to research at, inter alia,
- *Universite Laval* in Quebec City, Canada
- *University of Copenhagen* in Copenhagen, Denmark

To make a long story short, we should also mention

- **Eggs**

for support of weight management because of their rich content of vitamins (A&D), minerals (iron, calcium) as well as unsaturated fats and protein.

Scientifically verified by, inter alia, the *University of South Australia* in Adelaide, Australia.

IN A NUTSHELL

Being overweight or obese signals a susceptibility to various debilitating diseases. Therefore, it is crucial to be well-informed about nutrients to promote healthy weight management.

6. HEALTH – WHAT IS IT ALL ABOUT?

THE PHILOSOPHY BEHIND

Needless to stress that health is the overriding value of our physical/mental/social well-being – and longevity. That's why, according to the *Centers for Disease Control and Prevention (CDC)*, annual healthcare costs in the U.S. have crossed the mark of $3.5 trillion. With, inter alia, 1/3 of this amount for hospitalization, and 1/10 for prescription drugs.

Despite of that, however, the U.S. is ranking only 46 on *World Health Organization* global statistics of life expectancy. With special reference to broad spectrum of most debilitating but unsolved diseases as heart failure on top, followed by cancer. Despite of highly appreciated medical research and practice.

In fact, the philosophy behind of this vicious cycle is the necessity of appropriate lifestyle to tackle infirmities and threats endangering our daily life.

Basically, all factors contributing to our health are strongly linked and therefore, need to be balanced to achieve good health overall.

TYPES OF HEALTH – SCIENTIFICALLY VALIDATED

Based on research at, inter alia, the *Veterans Affairs Medical Center* in Tuscaloosa, Alabama.

For appropriate understanding, let's start with the respective types of health.

- **Physical health**

This type of health requires primarily a lifestyle cutting down the risk of developing certain diseases with respect to supporting physically the endurance of, inter alia,
    - heart function
    - breathing
    - body composition
    - muscular strength

- flexibility

with exercise, healthy diet and bodily rest.

By
- reducing risk of hazards at workplace
- avoiding tobacco and illegal drugs
- practicing appropriate hygiene
- etc.

This should well be in line with

- ***Mental health***

to be understood as the psychological, emotional and social well-being, as defined by the U.S. *Department of Health and Human Services.*

Thereby, mental health is not only an issue of depression and anxiety but also
- enjoying life
- balancing certain parts in life such as finances and family
- feeling safe/secure
- bouncing back when having difficult experiences
- adapting to adversity

In fact, there is a close relationship between physical and mental health especially in cases of chronic illness, leading manifold to stress and depression as the result of, inter alia, issues of mobility and/or financial problems.

FACTORS FOR GOOD HEALTH – SCIENTIFICALLY VALIDATED

While there are quite a few factors playing a role in our health, environment is one of most important, according the *World Health Organization (WHO).*

Based on research at, inter alia, the *University of Colorado* in Boulder, CO, and *Rice University* in Houston, TX.

In following terms:

- ***Physical environment***

Based on pollution in a certain area, with respective germs in place.

- ***Social/economic environment***

Potentially with respect to the respective quality of relationships and social culture in general, or the financial situation of family and/or community.

- ***Personal characteristics/behaviors***

With respect to the respective genetic pattern and lifestyle applied.

Research at, inter alia,
- *Yonsei University* in Wonju
- *Hankuk University of Foreign Studies* in Seoul
  &
- *Pai Chai University* in Daejeon
  (all 3 in South Korea)
  as well as
- *University of Kragujevac* in Kragujevac, Serbia

demonstrates that people with high socio-economic status afford good healthcare – and therefore better health.

Also, Dutch medical research at the
- *National Institute of Public Health and the Environment* in Bilthoven
  &
- *Wageningen University* in Wageningen

performed in European countries shows that *healthy diet* (with special reference to fruits, vegetables, and olives) lowered a 20-year death rate.

Similar the results of research at the *Grigore T. Popa University of Medicine and Pharmacy* in Lasi, Romania with respect to Mediterranean diet, with special reference to diabetes 2 and cancer.

Summing up briefly: the positive keyword is *wellness* to stay in good health, as demonstrated by the *World Health Organization*.

Covering, inter alia, following lifestyle aspects as indicated by, inter alia, the *American Heart Association*:
- balanced natural diet
- stress management
- exercising of 150 minutes per week (from moderate to high-intensity)
- see your future in a positive way

IN A NUTSHELL

Health is the most important value in our life, made up of our physical, mental and social well-being. To be well supported not only by its basic 2 pillars - physical exercise and healthy diet - but also additional lifestyle factors, as demonstrated above.

7. HOW AVERT BREAST CANCER NATURALLY

THE PHILOSOPHY BEHIND

Although breast cancer can basically hit both genders, in 99% of cases it is the most debilitating type of disease for women at all. According to research at, inter alia, *Turgut Özal University* in Ankara & *Fatih University* in Istanbul, both Turkey.

What's the cause – and how can we circumvent?

In fact, there are some factors we cannot circumvent. Like, inter alia,
- *family history*
  i.e. family members on mother's or father's side who had already breast cancer.
  Or inherited
- *genetic mutations*
  to specific genes like BRCA1/BRCA2.
  Also
- *dangerous medications*
  as those like diethylstilbestrol (DES) which had been prescribed between 1940 and 1971 to avoid miscarriage.
  Not to overlook
- *age*
  since most cases of cancer are diagnosed after age 50.

LIFESTYLE ADJUSTMENTS – SCIENTIFICALLY VALIDATED

Fortunately yet, there are well some lifestyle factors to ward off breast cancer, as briefly indicated in following.

Healthy diet

There are quite some foods to better limit or even avoid, like
- red/processed meat
- products of refined grain
  &
- sugary beverages

according to the *American Institute for Cancer Research* and the *World Cancer Research Fund.*

Instead, the *American Cancer Society,* the *U.S. Department of Agriculture* and *U.S. Department of Human Services* with the Advisory Committee of both, recommend in their Dietary Guidelines a diet high in

-    fruits
-    vegetables
-    whole grain

but at the same time low of

-    animal products
     &
-    refined carbohydrates

This is in line with a Mediterranean-type diet, adding olive oil, as based on research in Spain at, inter alia,

-    *University of Navarra-School of Medicine* in Pamplona
-    *Universitat Rovira I Virgili* in Reus
-    *University of Barcelona* in Barcelona
-    *University of Valencia* in Valencia
-    *University of Malaga* in Malaga
-    *Universitario Son Espases* in Palma de Mallorca
-    *University of Las Palmas de Gran Canaria* in Las Palmas

and in the U.S. at, inter alia,

-    *Harvard School of Public Health*
     &
-    *Harvard Medical School/Brigham and Women's Hospital*
     (both in Boston, MA)

Also, according to the above mentioned *American Institute for Cancer Research* and the *World Cancer Research Fund,* dairy products high in calcium (along with linoleic acid and Vitamin D) may help as well to prevent breast cancer.

Additional lifestyle factors

Based on the aforementioned *American Institute for Cancer Research* and the *World Cancer Research Fund,* following adjustments are also advisable in order to ward off breast cancer such as – inter alia -

- ### *Physical activity*

Practicing 75-150 minutes vigorous or 150 minutes moderate per week.

- ### *Body weight management*

Manage healthy body weight lifelong to avoid overweight/obesity.

This implies a

- ***Non-sedentary lifestyle***

To limit long periods of TV and other screen watching.

- ***Breastfeeding***

In cases of childbirth, breastfeeding is recommended, decreasing the risk of breast cancer later in life.

IN A NUTSHELL

Breast cancer is one of the most debilitating diseases for women at all. Still, it is not an ordeal, but can be turned down naturally at least to a certain degree. By appropriate lifestyle adjustments, as indicated above.

8. EATING RIGHT FOR YOUR HEALTH

THE PHILOSOPHY BEHIND

Needless to stress that nutrition is part of our health and existence at all. In terms of quantity and quality. Unfortunately yet, many of us do not match the biologic requirements of both. Leading to manifold – even debilitating – diseases and premature death. Just look at the statistics of the *World Health Organization (WHO)*, according to which 86% of non-age related premature death and 77% of all diseases in general are the consequence of unsolved health issues, at least in the industrialized countries. With special reference to unhealthy diet. The U.S. being no exception.

HEALTH-RELATED FACTORS – SCIENTIFICALLY VERIFIED

However, additionally to biologically appropriate nutrition, as we have covered quite a few times in our publications, our diet got to be embedded in an equally healthy lifestyle in general. This leaves us with the question which lifestyle factors shall be considered in this context.

Regular meal times

Besides of what we eat, the timely rhythm when we do so, is also of relevance for our health.

According to research at the *University of Nottingham* in Nottingham, UK, 6 regular meal times have not only a positive effect on our appetite and weight management but also on our metabolism in general.

Other than 3 to 9 irregular meal times.

Picking healthy diet

Needless to stress that our diet got to be healthy in lined with our biologic requirements.

Since we have covered a whole portfolio about healthy food, just let us pick one special:

- *apples*

Apples? You may know the saying 'An apple a day keeps the doctor away'. Because of its powerful antioxidants such as *quercetin* which, inter alia, is
-    supporting neurological health/turning down *dementia & Alzheimer's disease*

according to research in Colombia at the *University of Antioquia* in Medellin & *Universidad Nacional de Colombia* in Bogota.

Also it is
-    cutting down the risk of *stroke*

based on research at, inter alia, the *National University of Health Sciences* in Lombard, IL & the *University of Kuopio* in Kuopio, Finland.

As well as
-    lowering ('bad') *LDL cholesterol*

according to research at, inter alia, the *University of Copenhagen* in Frederiksberg, Denmark.

Not to forget about apple's power to
-    support heart health with its high content of vitamin C, fiber, and potassium.

Based on research at, inter alia, the *University of Connecticut* in Storrs, CT.

Even lowering risk of diabetes is part of apple's power. Based on research at, inter alia,
-    *Harvard School of Public Health* & *Harvard Medical School* in Boston, MA
-    *University of Cambridge* in Cambridge, UK
-    *National University of Singapore*

Finally
-    fighting cancer

according to research at the *University of Cambridge* in Cambridge, UK, with special reference to lung/breast/colorectal cancer.

Scientifically verified also by
-    *Southeast University* in Nanjing, China
     &
-    *Technical University* in Munich, Germany

Exercising

To exercise is releasing, inter alia, naturally so called 'feel good' chemicals in our brain regulating appetite and avoiding stress and anxiety – and overeating, accordingly.

According to research at, inter alia,
- *Abant Izzel Bay Sal University* in Bolu, Turkey
- *Lehman College* in West Bronx, NY
- *University of Texas Southwestern Medical Center* in Dallas, TX
- *Federal University of Rio Grande do Sul* in Porto Alegre, Brazil

Similar the situation when

Getting outside

At least once a day, preferably surrounded by nature, which is usually improving our mood. With the benefit of not to overeat.

Based on research at *Loyola University Chicago* in Maywood, IL

Stay hydrated

Staying hydrated during the day with plenty of drinking water especially already before meal may avoid overeating as well.

Based on research at, inter alia, *Jeonju University* in Jeonju, South Korea.

IN A NUTSHELL

Healthy diet is a basic pillar of our existence. Especially, if it is embedded in an equally healthy lifestyle pattern, as we have focused on in this chapter. Scientifically verified.

9. HEALTH BENEFITS OF GREEN LEAVY VEGGIES

THE PHILOSOPHY BEHIND

As you have learned from our previous scientifically validated publications, healthy diet – besides physical exercise – is one of basic warranties for health and longevity.

that's why the dietary guidelines of the U.S. Department of Agriculture (USDA) recommend that adults should fill at least half of their plate with fruits and vegetables.

With special reference to the edible plant leaves of certain vegetables because of the nutrients involved our body (and mind) needs. In order to support our immune system and self-healing power we can't replace with any synthetics.

So called green leafy vegetables (going also by the terms dark green leafy vegetables, leafy greens or simply greens) being in the forefront.

SPECIFIC TYPES FOR HEALTH – SCIENTIFICALLY VALIDATED

While there are many green leafy vegetables to be found in nature – and on the market, accordingly - we shall pick a couple of those in the following. To interpret their high content of nutrients and also fiber, and low content of calories, respectively. With special reference to those debilitating diseases ranking on top of World Health Organization (WHO) statistics of conventionally unsolved health problems: heart – cancer - diabetes.

SPINACH

This well-known veggie is a type of 'neuro-nutrition' which may help delay the onset of

- ***Alzheimer's Disease***

   Based on research at *Mahidol University* in Thailand's capital of Bangkok.

   With special reference to its content of, inter alia,

- protein 0.9 grams
   &
- fiber 0.7 grams

but only
- 7 calories
 in one cup (30 grams) of raw spinach.

According to U.S. Department of Agriculture.

CABBAGE

Like all cruciferous vegetables, also cabbage is rich in *sulforaphane*, which got the reputation to cut down the risk of

- ***cancer***

with special reference to *breast* cancer.

According to the U.S. *National Cancer Institute* in Bethesda/Frederick/Rockville, MD.

However, based on same research sulforaphane may also cut down the risk of

- ***stroke***

   &

- ***high blood pressure***

 with special reference to its content of
- protein 1.1 grams
- fiber 2.2. grams
   &
- calories 22
in one cup (89 grams) of chopped raw cabbage.

According to U.S. Department of Agriculture.

WATERCRESS

Also a cruciferous vegetable, watercress may help, inter alia, against

- ***chemotherapy damage***

and to prevent

- ***liver toxicity***

according to the U.S. *Centers for Disease Control and Prevention (CDC)*.

Containing, inter alia,
- protein 0.8 grams
- fiber 0.2 grams
  &
- calories 4
in one cup (34 grams) of raw watercress.

According to U.S. Department of Agriculture.

BOK CHOY

As a cruciferous vegetable as well it is helpful against

- ***infections***

according to the U.S. *National Institutes of Health (NIH)* because of its content of selenium.

Also containing
- protein 1.1 grams
- fiber 0.7 grams
  &
- calories 9
in one cup (70 grams) of shredded raw bok choy.

According to U.S. Department of Agriculture.

KALE

As a member of the cabbage family as well, its reputation is based, inter alia, on its high content of fiber and antioxidants to cut down the risk of

- ***diabetes 2***

according to research at the *National University of Health Sciences* in Lombard, IL.

With special reference to its content also of
- protein 3.5 grams
- fiber 4.7 grams
  &
- calories 43
in one cup (118 grams) of cooked kale.

According to U.S. Department of Agriculture.

ROMAINE LETTUCE

Based on its content of, inter alia, *beta carotene,* which is good for eye health, this type of lettuce may

- **prevent macular degeneration**

based on findings of the U.S. *National Institutes of Health (NIH).*

With special reference to its content of, inter alia,
- protein 0.6 grams
- fiber 1.0 grams
  &
- 8 calories
in one cup (47 grams) of shredded Romaine lettuce.

According to U.S. Department of Agriculture (USDA).

SWISS CHARD

This vegetable may

- **stop cancer growth**

  according to research at the

  - *University of Belgrade* in Belgrade, Serbia
    &
  - *University of Montenegro* in Podgorica, Montenegro.

With special reference to its content of
- protein 0.6 grams
- fiber 0.6 grams
   &
- 6.8 calories
in one cup (36 grams) of raw Swiss chard.

Also this based on USDA.

IN A NUTSHELL

According to the dietary guidelines of the U.S. Department of Agriculture (USDA) green leafy vegetables are of high relevance for our (physical and mental) health and longevity. To support our immune system and self-healing power in specific medical cases which we can't replace with any synthetics. In this chapter you learned more about in favor of your individual health.

10. HEALTHY & LONGER LIFE WITH NECTARINES?

THE PHILOSOPHY BEHIND

As you have learned, inter alia, from my previous publications, our health depends, besides physical exercise, on natural diet with special reference to fruits and vegetables.

For better understanding, let's focus on one specific fruit – nectarines.

NATURAL MEDICAL BENEFITS – SCIENTIFICALLY VALIDATED

The nutritional background of this favorite fruit comes with a range of health benefits. Just to pick some of those, according to the U.S. *Department of Agriculture.*

Cutting down high blood pressure

Potassium as one of the basic constituents in nectarines, it is an excellent support to keep blood pressure under control, since hypertension hurts prime organs like our heart. With special reference to heart attack, coronary heart disease and stroke. According to the U.S. *Centers for Disease Control and Prevention (CDC).*

As based also on research at, inter alia, the *Hypertension Institute* in Nashville, TN.

Strengthen immune system

Based on the fact that there is infection behind any disease, *vitamin C* (as we find it, inter alia, in nectarines) tackles this risk considerably.

According to research at, inter alia, the *University of Otago* in Christchurch, New Zealand.

Therefore, the scientists recommend an increased intake of vitamin C rich food. Especially in Western countries where populations are lacking appropriate amount of this vital vitamin.

Saving skin health

Also *vitamin A* is important, as we find it in nectarines, supporting our skin health by saving it from UV radiation.

The mineral *copper* on the other hand, also to be found in nectarines, supports the elasticity of our skin.

According to research at, inter alia, *Jan Kochanowski University* in Kielce, Poland.

Weight management

The benefit of nectarines for weight control lies, inter alia, on the fact that they are sweet but low in fat and calories. Also helpful is their content of *fiber* which offers quick saturation without overeating.

According to, inter alia, the U.S. *Centers for Disease Control and Prevention (CDC)*.

Cancer prevention

One of the powerful phytonutrients in nectarines are *anthocyanins* which are known for their anti-tumor properties of being
- anti-inflammatory
- antioxidant
  &
- mutation-preventing

That's why, according to the *Tongji University School of Medicine* in Shanghai, China, these anthocyanins may well represent an anti-cancer power.

This is also in line with the results of research at the *Kyoto Prefectural University of Medicine* in Kyoto, Japan, according to which cancer has an inverse relation to the consumption of green and yellow fruits and vegetables.

Even more than that:

Support longevity

Built on research at the U.S. *National Institute of Aging* in Baltimore, MD,
- *Harvard School of Public Health* in Boston, MA,
  along with
- *Huazhong University of Science and Technology* in Wuhan,
  &
- *Shandong University* in Jinan
  (both China)

came to the scientific conclusion that
- *higher consumption of fruits and vegetables may well*
- *lower the risk of mortality from all causes.*

IN A NUTSHELL

Fruits, like vegetables, are of great value for a healthy and long life. Based on their specific nutritional content. Just look at nectarines as one example. Scientifically validated.

11. WALK OFF POOR HEALTH & MORTALITY?

THE PHILOSOPHY BEHIND

As you have learned from our previous publications, physical exercise is a basic prerequisite for good health and longevity.

With tremendous effects on our physical and mental wellbeing, as indicated by the U.S. *Centers for Disease Control and Prevention (CDC)*. Such as, inter alia,
- sound sleep quality
- cutting down the risk of anxiety and depression
- improving memory capacity
- supporting muscles and bones

More than that: according to same CDC source, it may also reduce the risk of those 3 most debilitating health issues in our seemingly modern society, based on statistics of the *World Health Organization (WHO):*
- heart failure
- cancer
- diabetes

COUNT YOUR DAILY STEPS – SCIENTIFICALLY VERIFIED

This medical benefit comes with special reference to walking at least 7000 steps per day. With the number of steps counting more than their intensity.

Along with lowering the risk of premature mortality.

Scientifically supported in the U.S. by, inter alia,
- *National Cancer Institute* in Rockville, MD
- *National Center for Chronic Disease Prevention and Health Promotion* in Atlanta, GA
- *National Institute of Aging* in Bethesda, MD
  &
- *University of Tennessee* in Knoxville, TN

With scientific verification also by *Coronary Artery Risk Development in Young Adults (CARDIA)* at the *University of Alabama* in Birmingham, AL, with chapters at

- *University of Minnesota* in Minneapolis, MN
- *Oakland Clinical Center* in Oakland, CA
- *Northwestern University* in Chicago, IL

As well as by international research at, inter alia,
- *Umea University* in Umea, Sweden
- *Arctic University* in Tromso, Norway
- *University College Cork* in Cork, Ireland
- *Ulster University* in Londonderry, UK
- *Karelia University of Applied Sciences* in Joensuu, Finland

This implies, however, to control potentially counterproductive health issues such as, inter alia,

- high blood pressure
- high body mass index (overweight/obesity)
- smoking
- high cholesterol & blood glucose levels
- high alcohol intake
- medications

IN A NUTSHELL

Physical activity, besides healthy diet, is one of the prime pillars for sound health and longevity. With special reference also to the most debilitating health issues (according to WHO statistics) such as heart failure, cancer and diabetes – and premature mortality. Provided, you walk at least 7000 steps daily according to scientific verification, as focused on in this chapter.

12. SOCIAL IMPLICATIONS OF YOUR HEALTH?

THE PHILOSOPHY BEHIND

As you have learned, inter alia, from our previous publications, the 2 pillars carrying sound health are appropriate diet and physical exercise. Leaves us with the question, on which fundament these 2 pillars are resting on.

SOCIAL LIFESTYLE FACTORS – SCIENTIFICALLY VERIFIED

Eating and moving our body right requires appropriate circumstances in daily life we may not want to overlook from a life-long socioeconomic, political and cultural perspective. Such as where and when being born, growing up, live, work, and age. With special reference to those social circumstances surrounding us in our contemporary daily life.

According to the *World Health Organization (WHO)*.

I.e., taking care of ourselves just medically covers not more than 10-20% of our health situation according to the U.S. *National Academy of Medicine*. For the balance (80-90%) social implications are responsible, like the following.

Economic stability

...is overall important to finance not only appropriate medical treatment but also to support different lifestyle factors, healthy diet included.

According to the *Office of Disease Prevention and Health Promotion* at the U.S. *Department of Health and Human Services (ODPHP)*.

In fact, life expectancy of those living in countries with appropriate economic stability is skyrocketing by 19 years, according to the *World Health Organization (WHO)*.

Unfortunately yet, 10% of the U.S. population live in poverty, according to the U.S. *Department of Commerce*.

That's why *ODPHP* has launched a program named *Healthy People 2030* with focus on
- career counseling

- employment programs
  &
- high quality child care

To support citizens in need to pay not only for appropriate healthcare but complementary for appropriate (health-related)
- food
- education
  &
- housing

Sound education

According to research at the *University of California* in San Francisco, CA, data from the U.S. and Europe indicate that there is indeed a strong relationship between health status and education based on individual income. Especially as people may not get an appropriate education already at young age and beyond, lacking appropriate funds.

Leading finally to heart disease, diabetes and depression in many cases. Aggravated by stress.

As supported also by *ODPHP*.

Social relationships

Getting together with family members and colleagues at workplace does also have an impact on health, according to *ODPHP*. With special reference to our mood and self-esteem – both an impact on health. In good or bad, depending on the quality of this relationship. Not to overlook that a lack of social interactions at all may lead to the feeling of loneliness with impact on our health, accordingly. For kids and adults alike.

To avoid or overcome negative situations, the above mentioned *Healthy People 2030* campaign helps by supporting social care and activities, thus reducing also depression and anxiety. Especially for kids and folks with disabilities, who are lacking manifold social contacts otherwise.

Environmental surroundings

It is manifold underestimated how many people live in crime-ridden and environmentally disturbed areas with – yes – a direct impact on their health.

Not only in their private sphere but also at work (e.g., when affected by secondhand smoke, just to mention one example).

With less chance to overcome at least in outdoor cases where public economic impact plays a role.

It is easier to react indoor in favor of a toxin-free environment in cases of, inter alia,
- tobacco smoke
- household chemicals
- mold
  or
- certain building materials (such as asbestos or lead, etc.)
according to the *World Health Organization (WHO).*

IN A NUTSHELL

Healthy diet and physical activity are certainly the basic pillars of or existence. However, they need to be fundamentally supported by certain lifestyle factors. That's almost common knowledge by now. But: there is new research and evidence to back this, as you have learned in this chapter.

13. WHY & HOW HANDLE DIABETES NATURALLY?

THE PHILOSOPHY BEHIND

The conventional medical system in our industrialized world – with special reference to the U.S. – is most advanced in history. Honored with 9 out of 10 Nobel Prizes in medicine.

Still, according to the World Health Organization (WHO), 86% of non-age-related deaths and 77% of all ailments in general are the consequence of some 1800 – mostly preventable – chronic diseases. With diabetes 2 on top of the chart, just behind heart failure and cancer, as a progressive disease, cutting life expectancy by 10 years potentially.

With following symptoms many pre-diabetics may not be fully aware as, inter alia:
- tingling/numbness in hands/feet
- increase of thirst/urination
- dry skin
- tiredness
- increased feeling of hunger
- blurry vision
- slow healing of sores
- increase of infections

Although the U.S. is spending most per capita for medicine globally.

Just take the worldwide mostly prescribed drug for diabetes which, according to its producer (pharma giant *Bristol Myers Squibb*) comes with more than 80 side effects – but no cure.

NATURE'S WAY OUT OF VICIOUS CYCLE – VERIFIED BY SCIENCE

Instead, scientific research at, inter alia, the *University of Laval* in Quebec City, Canada, supported by the *American Diabetic Association (ADA)* is pointing at a natural way out based on certain healthy lifestyle practices. Let's focus on 5 of those, as follows.

Healthy diet

In line with the basics of Mediterranean diet, the *American Diabetic Association (ADA)*, along with the *Dietary Guidelines for Americans* of the

U.S. Department of Agriculture, recommends nutritious consumption of, inter alia,
- whole grains

like brown rice/oatmeal/whole grain bread/ whole-wheat or legume pasta/wild rice/cornmeal/barley/oatmeal/amaranth/millet/100% whole grain-whole wheat flour/quinoa.

Also
- fruits (with special reference to apples/oranges/cherries/apricots pears/peaches/grapefruit, etc.)

As well as
- vegetables (such as broccoli/Brussel sprouts/cauliflower/green beans/red-yellow-orange peppers/squash/onions/asparagus/salad greens).

Plus
- olive oil
- fatty fish rich in omega-3 fatty acids like non-fried salmon/lake trout
- nuts & seeds (unsalted)
- legumes (like peas/beans/ black beans/white beans/lentils/chickpeas/kidney beans/pinto beans)
- dairy (such as cottage cheese/ricotta/Parmesan/plain yogurt/low fat or fat free Greek yogurt/skimmed or low-fat milk
- low fat fish
- lean meat (such as sirloin/white meat from chicken/turkey)
- protein-rich food (like eggs/tuna/tofu/tempeh/skinless-boneless chicken breasts or strips/white fish filets/tofu/tempeh/sardines/skinless turkey breast)

...to control blood sugar.

Scientifically supported by the
- *University of Granada* in Granada
  &
- *Hospital del Mar Medical Research Institute* in Barcelona (both Spain)

Vice-versa, (pre-)diabetics may refrain from following foods. Inter alia,
- processed and fatty meats, such as bacon, hot dogs, and fatty cuts of beef and pork
- salty foods
- saturated fat like foods containing coconut oil or palm oil

- partially hydrogenated and trans fat foods like shortening/ hard margarine/microwave popcorn/frozen pizzas,/desserts/ coffee creamer
- sweet food additives like high fructose corn syrup//dextrose/maltose, fructose, and sucrose additives, such as high fructose corn syrup, dextrose, maltose, fructose, and sucrose
- sugary foods and beverages like candy/cakes/jelly/honey/sodas/sweet tea/fruit drinks/concentrated fruit juices

Healthy diet has also the benefit of weight management which plays a major role in cases of diabetes. Equally as – and this is the next lifestyle factor to focus on to handle diabetes naturally –

Physical exercise

As it helps with the management of blood sugar by supporting insulin sensitivity not to let blood sugar enter cells from bloodstream.

According to research at
-   *School of Allied Health Sciences*
    &
-   *Kasturba Medical College*
    (both in Manipal, India)

Along with the recommendation to exercise moderately 150 minutes (or vigorously 75 minutes) per week. Regularly.

As an additional positive side effect, both – healthy diet and regular (preferably aerobic) exercise - also help with ...

Weight management

... which is promoting also management of blood sugar by consuming less calories.

According to *Newcastle University* in Newcastle upon Tyne, UK, practicing weight management for 12 months may well cut down diabetes.

Stress management

While stress by itself does not lead to diabetes 2, it may well worsen it, hampering regulation of blood sugar.

According to research at, inter alia,

- *Avalon University School of Medicine* in Girard, OH
  &
- *California Institute of Behavioral Neurosciences and Psychology* in Fairfield, CA

To avoid stress, the *American Heart Association (AHA)* recommends, inter alia, to relax in nature.

Also

Non-smoking

is important when it comes to manage blood sugar, since smoking increases the risk of diabetes by roughly one third.

Along with the risk to also develop nerve damage and/or kidney disease as an additional negative side effect.

IN A NUTSHELL

According to the World Health Organization (WHO), diabetes 2 is one of the leading and most debilitating chronic diseases of our time. Cutting down our life expectancy, with premature, non-age-related death in many cases. Without conventional medical solution so far. That's why the American Diabetic Association (ADA) recommends nature for the way out, as you have learned in this chapter.

14. KNOW HEALTH BENEFIT OF FRUIT JUICES?

THE PHILOSOPHY BEHIND

As you have learned from our previous publications, fruits belong to the most beneficial nutrition to support our health and longevity. With special reference to those diseases leading the premature, non-age-related death toll statistics of the World Health Organization (WHO): cardiovascular disease, cancer and diabetes.

Regardless, if the fruits are consumed in whole or as a juice. Although it is more beneficial to eat whole fruit, fruit juices are certainly of nutritional advantage as well and which we may not want to overlook.

At least, as long as we avoid overconsumption which could lead to weight gain or harm your blood sugar level.

In this respect, especially children may limit their fruit juice consumption because of high amounts of sugar involved.

According to research at, inter alia,
- *Chonbuk National University* in Jeonju
  &
- *Seonam University* in Namwon

(both South Korea)

This implies that children 1-3 years old may consume per day no more than 4 ounces of fruit juice, at age 4-6 limit to 4-6 ounces, and up to 8 ounces at age 7 and beyond.

Not only children. Consuming too much fruit juices may lead, e.g., also to *diabetes* in cases of adults, according to research at, inter alia,
- *Shandong University* in Jinan, China
  &
- *University of Minnesota* in Minneapolis, MN.

However, the real problem with fruits (and vegetables) is rather that 90% of our adults do not eat enough fruits and the respective nutrients in it.

I.e. males should consume at least 2 cups of fruit per day, females at least 1 and a half.

According to the *Behavioral Risk Factor Surveillance System* of the U.S. *Centers for Disease Control and Prevention (CDC)*.

Just let's focus on the benefits of certain fruit juices in following.

Cranberry juice

This fruit juice may help comprehensively in cases of, inter alia,
- *high blood pressure*
- *inflammation*
- *cholesterol*
- *glucose metabolism*
  and
- *oxidative stress*

According to international research at, inter alia,
- *Pennsylvania State University* at University Park, PA
- *Heinrich-Heine-University* in Düsseldorf, Germany
- *University of East Anglia* in Norwich, UK
- *Rutgers University* in Chatsworth, NJ
  as well as
- *Boston University*
  &
- *Tufts University*
  (both in Boston, MA)

With the additional benefit of cutting the risk of

- *urinary tract infection*

Based on research at *Universidade da Beira Interior* in Covilha, Portugal

Orange juice

The great value of this type of fruit juice is certainly its content of *vitamin C.* By reducing following health issues according to the U.S. *National Institutes of Health (NIH):*
- *cardiovascular disease*
- *cancer*
- *eye disease* (cataracts & macular degeneration – AMD)
- *common cold*

Another beneficial component of orange juice is vitamin B-9 (folate), supporting
- *fetal development and growth.*

According to *NIH* as well.

Tomato juice

Unlike manifold folk wisdom, however, tomatoes are not vegetables but, yes, they are *fruits.*

However, their health benefit are not only their high content of *vitamin C* like orange juice (as indicated above).

The additional high content of *lycopene* helps to reduce

- *cardiovascular disease*

According to *Zhengzhou University* in Zhengzhou, China.

Not enough. Also *potassium*, a beneficial component of tomato juice as well, helps with *reducing blood pressure,* and the risk of *stroke* and *heart disease.*

According to the U.S. *Centers for Disease Control and Prevention (CDC).*

Pomegranate juice

This type of fruit juice, on the other hand, is a powerful source of *vitamin K* supporting our *heart.*

Based on comprehensive medical research in The Netherlands at the
- *Vrije Universiteit Amsterdam*
  &
- *VU University Medical Center*
  (also Amsterdam)
  as well as the
- *University Medical Center Utrecht* in Utrecht

Additionally, *vitamin K* supports *memory* especially in older people, according to research at the *University of Montreal* in Montreal, Canada.

IN A NUTSHELL

Healthy diet is one of the vital basics of our health and longevity. With special reference to fruits and their inherent nutrients. Regardless, if consumed in whole or as a juice. In this chapter you learn about the health benefits of some fruit juices you may not want to miss.

15. WHICH FOODS TO MIND FOR BETTER SLEEP?

THE PHILOSOPHY BEHIND

Needless to stress that sound sleep is vital to relax and strengthen body and mind.

Unfortunately yet, according to Australian research at
- *Central Queensland University* in Melbourne
  &
- *Griffith University* at Gold Coast

almost half of the adult population in Australia and the U.S. don't get 7-9 hours of sound sleep per day to fulfill this prerequisite.

Not only this. One third of the U.S. population are suffering insomnia, i.e. having difficulty to fall asleep and to prolong good quality sleep.

According to research at the *University of Missouri* in Columbia, MS.

The philosophy behind, however, is not only based on mental irregularities or physical problems like pain, even certain/inappropriate nutrition may well play a role in this context.

SLEEP HAMPERING FOODS – SCIENTIFICALLY VERIFIED

In fact, there are foods hampering sound sleep, we may want to control. Such as, inter alia...

- ### *Spicy foods*

...causing, inter alia, heartburn, rise of temperature, acid reflux, and indigestion which may well disturb our sleep.

Based on research at *Ziauddin University Hospital* in Karachi, Pakistan.

- ### *Processed foods*

...like industrially prepackaged and so called 'fast' food) with manifold high amounts of fats and sugars. With a negative impact on our sleep as well by promoting indigestion.

According to research at, inter alia, *Universidade Federal do Maranhao* in Maranhao, Brazil.

Also for young people aged 12-18, based on research at
- *Seoul National University* in Seoul
  &
- *Hallym University College of Medicine* in Anyang
  (both South Korea)

- **Fatty foods/saturated fats**

...like desserts and fatty meats being also responsible for acid reflux and indigestion.

According to international research at
- *Ziauddin University Hospital* in Karachi, Pakistan
  &
- *Columbia University* in New York, NY.

- **Sugary foods**

(also called high glycemic foods) like potatoes/white rice/candy.

Based on research at, inter alia, *Capital Medical University* in China's capital Beijing.

Not to overlook

- **Caffeine**

...which is stimulating your central nervous system.

And as it is part not only in coffee but also part of , inter alia,
- tea
- soda/cola
- energy drinks
  &
- chocolate

With the negative effect of
- not falling asleep in time
- cutting down sleep quality & sleep time
- increasing arousals & wakefulness.

According to research at, inter alia, the *University of Zurich* in Zurich, Switzerland.

Potentially creating symptoms like, inter alia,
- rapid heartbeat
- insomnia
- headaches
- restlessness
- nausea
- dizziness
- dehydration
- anxiety

According to the U.S. *Centers for Disease Control and Prevention (CDC)*.

That's why the U.S. *Food and Drug Administration (FDA)* recommends to limit daily coffee consumption with 4-5 cups.

Unless you have reason to, stay awake for whatsoever.

Also

- ● ***Alcohol***

as it may turn out problematic as a depressant and therefore, does not support sound sleep.

Especially, as it interferes with our *circadian rhythm* and therefore worsens quality of our sleep

According to *London Sleep Centre-Neuropsychiatry* in UK's capital London.

That's why the U.S. *Centers for Disease Control and Prevention (CDC)* recommend to refrain from alcohol before bed.

IN A NUTSHELL

There are different mental and physical implications to miss sound sleep. Not only. Rather, there are also certain foods interfering with, and interrupting with healthy sleep. As you have learned about in this chapter.

16. APPROPRIATE NUTRITION FOR DIABETICS?

THE PHILOSOPHY BEHIND

As you have learned from our multiple publications, diabetes is
- one of the top debilitating diseases in our 'modern' society
- with no conventional medical solution yet.

The more, it is important to manage this vicious cycle in line with nature. In order to balancing low and high glycemic index (speak: the blood sugar level) best. Especially in terms of daily diet.

NUTRITIONAL CATEGORIZATION – SCIENTIFICALLY SUPPORTED

To be on the safe side in this respect, let us be guided by following examples of the U.S. Department of Agriculture, supported by multiple international medical research.

Let's start with

Berries

such as...

- blackberries
- raspberries
- blueberries
- strawberries

being loaded with antioxidants preventing *oxidative stress*, leading potentially to many different diseases. Since oxidative stress is also highly common in many cases of diabetes, berries can counterbalance in this case.

Besides of the fact that berries are also rich in vitally important nutrients like
- vitamins C&K
- potassium
  &
- manganese

According to research at the *University of Arizona* in Tucson, AZ.

Citrus fruits

Like lemons, oranges and grapefruits are equally powerful in cases of diabetes.

As they contain 2 powerful bioflavonoid antioxidants (hesperidin & naringin) because of their strong antidiabetic effect – especially oranges.

Additionally to their nutrient content of
- folate
- vitamin c
  &
- potassium

Based on research at *Zhejiang University* in Hangzhou, China.

Sweet potatoes

have an even lower glycemic index (GI) than white potatoes and therefore are not raising blood sugar extensively and release sugar slowly..

Therefore, they are favorite of the *American Diabetic Association*.

With the additional benefit of containing
- vitamin A&C
- potassium
  &
- fiber

Also

Beans

with their species of
- black
- adzuki
- pinto
- kidney
  &
- navy

beans are helpful for diabetics in terms of regulating blood sugar, being low on glycemic index (GI).

According to research at *North Dakota State University* in Fargo, ND.

Additionally, they are helpful with weight loss and blood pressure as well as cholesterol regulation.

Chia seeds

have the benefits of helping to lose weight specifically in cases of overweight diabetics.

Also containing
- plant-based protein
  &
- fiber

Based on international research at, inter alia,
- *University of Toronto* in Toronto, Canada
  &
- *University of Zagreb* in Zagreb, Croatia.

Probiotic yogurt

has been identified scientifically to lower cholesterol level in diabetics.

According to research at, inter alia, *Tabriz University* in Tabriz, Iran.

Based on an additional research at *Universidade Federal de Goias* in Goias, Brazil, probiotic yogurt may also cut down oxidative stress and inflammation, thus increasing insulin sensitivity.

Whole grains

There are some medical facts in favor of whole grain to be considered in relation to diabetes.

One central argument is its content of fiber as it is slowing down the nutritional absorption, thus stabilizing the level of blood sugar.

At the same time, their glycemic index (GI) is also lower which means that there is no negative impact on blood sugar involved.

Accordingly, the *American Diabetic Association (ADA)* recommends, inter alia, following whole grains to consume for diabetics:
- rye
- buckwheat
- brown rice

- quinoa
- whole grain bread/pasta
- bulgur
- millet

Avoiding white bread/pasta at the same time.

Green leafy vegetables

Such as
- spinach
- cabbage
- broccoli
- bok choy
- kale
  &
- collard greens

are beneficial for diabetics not only because of their content of antibiotics but also their starch-digesting enzymes.

According to research at, inter alia, the *CSIR-Indian Institute of Chemical Technology* in Hyderabad, India.

Even more than that. Consuming 300 ml kale juice per day for 6 weeks may support regulation of blood sugar (and blood pressure).

Based on research at *Hannam University* in Daejeon, South Korea.

Walnuts

According to research at the *University of California* in Los Angeles, CA, the consumption of walnuts may well help to fight diabetes.

Not to forget about ...

Fatty fish

According to the *American Diabetic Association (ADA),* mono- & polyunsaturated fats are beneficial for control of blood sugar.

Therefore, it is certainly beneficial for diabetics to consume this type of fish such as, inter alia,
- mackerel
- salmon

- trout
- herring
- sardines
  &
- albacore tuna

Plus or alternatively seaweed (like spirulina and kelp).

Finally,
- *Harvard Medical School*
  &
- *Tufts University*
  (both in Boston, MA)
recommend...

Mediterranean diet

with eating less red meat but more healthy fats and vegetables instead. The researchers noted that this diet improved fasting plasma glucose and insulin levels among study participants.

On the other hand, diabetics may limit nutrition with high glycemic index (GI) such as, inter alia.
- white bread/pasta/rice/potatoes
- puffed rice
- popcorn
- pineapple
  &
- pumpkin

Above all, diabetics may refrain from

- refined sugar

as far as possible.

As also recommended by the *American Heart Association (AHA),* women may consume no more than 24 grams (6 teaspoons) and men no more than 36 grams (9 teaspoons) of industrially refined/added sugar per day.

At the same time, the *American Diabetes Association (ADA)* recommends to limit daily salt/sodium intake to less than 2,300 milligram per person. Regardless of diabetic status.

IN A NUTSHELL

Most importantly, it is vital for diabetics to manage blood sugar - speak: balance low and high glycemic index (GI) best. To do so, diet plays a decisive role. I.e. picking the appropriate daily nutrients. Like those indicated in this chapter.

17. SWALLOW HEADACHE NATURALLY?

THE PHILOSOPHY BEHIND

Headache is a highly prevalent health issue in our 'modern' society. Either as a primary case, i.e. with no other medical problem involved, or secondary as the consequence (symptom) of an underlying physical or mental cause.

According to the *International Headache Society (HIS)* in London, UK, we differ basically between 4 types of headaches (with varying pain intensity/severity):

- *Tension-type headache* - also named *stress headache* (causing mild/moderate dull pain)
- *Sinus headache* (secondary headache – due to buildup of pressure from inflammation)
- *Cluster headache* (usually on one side of head/around one eye, causing intense pain)
- *Migraine* (either in one area or on side of the head/neck, also with intense pain)

In most cases being pushed away with a pill, either way. That's it? If there were not quite a few side effects involved – a vicious cycle...

As you have learned from our previous publications, fortunately there are herbs and lifestyle adjustments to tackle the situation naturally.

HEADACHE-REPELLENT DIET – SCIENTIFICALLY VERIFIED

Not only. Recent scientific findings demonstrate that there is also some kind of nutrition waiving headache as well and which you may not want to miss. As you will find out in following.

Fruits/vegetables

With special reference to
- berries (like blue-/straw-/raspberries)

- bright-colored vegetables (like carrots/bell peppers)
- root vegetables (like beets/sweet potatoes)
- mushrooms (like maitake/shitake/oyster)
- spicy peppers (like cayenne)
- leafy green vegetables (like spinach/chard/kale)
- spices (like ginger/turmeric/garlic)

Based on the fact that they contain many antioxidants which are reducing oxidative stress & are fighting against free radical damage.

With the benefit of treating/preventing headache pain - especially *migraines*.

According to research at, inter alia, *Pomeranian Medical University* in Szczecin, Poland.

Also, research at *California State University* in Hayward, CA, concluded that a low-fat/high fiber diet with plant foods only may relieve migraine symptoms.

Water

Staying hydrated is not only important for health basically.

It may reduce or even prevent headache pain specifically. According to research in the UK at *University of Oxford* in Oxford & *City University London*.

Caffeinated foods

Since blood vessels tend to enlarge before headache strikes, *moderate* consumption of caffeine may constrict them because of its vasoconstrictive property, thus easing headache symptoms.

According to the U.S. *National Headache Foundation* in Chicago, IL.

Which caffeine-containing foods to consider in this case? Besides coffee, inter alia,
- green/black tea
- chocolate

In this context, we may also not to overlook...

Herbal teas

...which are not only hydrating but also may contain pain-relieving properties.

E.g., *ginger* tea has proven to relieve severe *migraine*, according to research at *Zanjan University of Medical Sciences* in Zanjan, Iran.

Also *chamomile* tea may relieve *tension headache*.

According to the U.S. *National Center for Complementary and Integrative Health (NCCIH)*.

Just as there is also food on the market being counterproductive in terms of headache and which we better mind.

On the other hand, there are...

FOODS POTENTIALLY TRIGGERING HEADACHE

...or worsen it because of specific additives involved. Such as
- aspartame
- sulfites
- nitrites
  &
- monosodium glutamate (MSG)

Just to name a few MSG-related examples:

- fast food (e.g. fried chicken/burgers, etc.)
- snacks (e.g. potato chips)
- frozen/processed meals/meats (e.g. sausages/bacons/hamburgers, etc.)
- sauces/dressings (e.g. barbecue/soy sauce, salad dressings)

As based on research at, inter alia, the *University of Tokyo* in Japan's capital.

IN A NUTSHELL

While there are herbs and lifestyle factors to tackle headache naturally (as you have learned in our previous publications), international science has also identified specific foods going into this direction, as we have indicated in this chapter.

18. FIGHTING CANCER WITH TROPICAL HERBS?

THE PHILOSOPHY BEHIND

The U.S. is foremost in conventional medicine, honored with 9 out of 10 Nobel prizes in this field of competence. Spending most per capita for medicine in the industrialized world.

Still, according to World Health Organization (WHO) statistics, 86% of non-age-related premature deaths are the consequence of unsolved ('chronic') health problems - with cancer on top. That fuels the efforts of research to find a way out of this vicious circle. And that is true for natural medicine as well. There are various recent studies on herbs with encouraging results in terms of cancer.

TROPICAL ANTI-CANCER HERBS - SCIENTIFICALLY VALIDATED

Some 20% of inhabitants develop cancer as the prime cause of premature death also in the Asian country of Singapore. That's why researchers at renowned University of Singapore have investigated some herbs, i.e. extracts of leaves from following plants native to South Asia (botanical names in brackets):

- *Fool's Curry Leaf (clausena lansium)*
- *Black Face General (strobilanthes crispus)*
- *Sabah Snake Grass (clinacanthus nutans)*
- *Seven Star Needle (pereskia bleo)*
- *Bandicoot Berry (leea indica)*
- *South African Leaf (vernonia amygdalina)*
- *Simpleleaf Chastetree (vitex trifolia)*

Specifically with respect to following types of cancer:
- colon
- breast
- uterine
- liver
- ovarian
- cervical
  &
- leukemia

Although these herbs have been known because of their medicinal effect for centuries, cancer was basically a new challenge.
As a result,

- South African leaf
- bandicoot Berry
  &
- simpleleaf chasetree

demonstrated powerful against all these cancers

Additionally,

- black face general
  as well as
- fool's curry

were at least efficient against some of these cancer types.

The only inefficient plant in terms of cancer was Sabah Snake Grass.

Another research has been carried out – in favor of esophageal cancer – internationally by, inter alia,
- *University of Mauritius* in Reduit, Mauritius
  &
- *University of Edinburgh* in Edinburgh
- *Keele University* in Keele
  (both UK)
  as well as
- *Far Eastern Federal University* in Vladivostok, Russia

Based on tropical herbs

- acalypha integrifolia
- eugenia tinifolia
  &
- labourdonnaisia glauca

which are native (only) to the island of Mauritius with one third of local plants being used for medicinal purposes since ancient times.

With the result that these medicinal herbs have demonstrated successful also in this case.

IN A NUTSHELL

Cancer is still one of the most premature deaths. That fuels the efforts of research to find a way out of this vicious circle. And that is true for natural medicine as well. There are various recent studies on herbs with encouraging results in terms of cancer. As you have learned in this chapter.

19. NATURAL SUPPORT FOR ARTHRITIS RELIEF

THE PHILOSOPHY BEHIND

According to the U.S. *Centers for Disease Control and Prevention,* some 60 million U.S. adults are suffering from stiffening and painful joints, and surrounding areas. Cutting down their wellbeing drastically in daily life.

While synthetic medicine has not offered a satisfactory solution, there are, however, some natural answers to relieve this debilitating chronic disease we may not want to overlook. With special reference to rheumatoid arthritis (RA) & osteoarthritis (OA).

NATURAL REMEDIES – SCIENTIFICALLY VERIFIED

Based on latest international research, inter alia, in Sweden at
- *Stockholm University* in Stockholm
  &
- *University of Gothenburg* in Gothenburg

as well as the
- *University of Oslo* in Norway's capital Oslo,

we learn about highly beneficial nutrients to tackle arthritis naturally.

Just to name 3 of those with anti-inflammatory power:

Curcumin

As you may remember from our seminar *Health from the Bible*, the 3 Wise Men offered 3 most powerful medicinal herbs to Jesus' birth, as documented already in the Holy Bible 2000 years ago. With *curcumin* (the basic part of glorious herb *turmeric*) – being one of those. In order to fight inflammation which is underlying any disease – arthritis being no exception.

Now we understand from traditional Chinese medical practice at, inter alia,
- *Dongying People's Hospital* in Dongying
  &
- *Nanjing Jinling Hospital* in Nanjing
  (both People's Republic of China)

that this herb is also a very effective remedy to fight rheumatoid arthritis (RA).

Even more. As it is scientifically verified in Australia, it fights also osteoarthritis (OA) according to the
- *University of Tasmania* in Tasmania
- *University of Queensland* in Brisbane
- *Monash University* in Melbourne
  &
- *Royal Hobart Hospital* in Hobart

As another biblical herb of the 3 holy remedies documented in the Holy Script by the 3 Wise Men, also

Boswellia

(the Indian herb *frankincense*) has been scientifically verified being powerful for rheumatoid arthritis according, inter alia, *King Georgia's Medical University* in Lucknow, India.

Not only. Also as a powerful remedy for osteoarthritis (OA), according to research in the People's Republic of China at
- *Guilin Medical University* in Guilin
- *University of South China* in Hengyang
- *Chinese Academy of Medical Sciences*
  &
- *Peking Union Medical College*
  (both in China's capital Beijing)
- *Hunan University of Chinese Medicine* in Changsha
- *People's Hospital of Ningxiang City* in Ningxian

Fish oil

In this case, the benefit for arthritis relief is certainly its content of anti-inflammatory omega-3 fatty acids in fish oil. Just to take low dose of it.

According to research at the *State University of Maringa* in Maringa, Brazil. With special reference to osteoarthritis (OA).

IN A NUTSHELL

Arthritis – the debilitating stiffness and pain of joints and surrounding areas in our body – has struck some 60 million adults in the U.S. alone. Fortunately, nature offers us relief with some special remedies.

20. HOW RELIEVE HOLIDAY GERD NATURALLY?

THE PHILOSOPHY BEHIND

I am sure you enjoy your family reunions like on Thanksgiving & X-mas along with the food you share. Hopefully without 'heartburn', a type of (diet-related) *acid reflux* in middle of the chest along with pain in the upper abdomen. Known by the medical term *gastroesophageal reflux* (GER) and GERD+ - the D standing for 'disease' in cases where it happens more than twice a week.

Based on symptoms like, inter alia,
- sore throat
- food regurgitation
- wheezing/weak coughing
- hoarseness or other changes to voice
- burping
- hiccups

Unfortunately, 20% of adults in the industrialized part of the world – like ours - are affected by GER/D.

According to
- *Johns Hopkins Hospital* in Tampa, FL
- *Homestead Hospital* in Homestead, FL
  &
- *Lehigh Valley Network* in Allentown, PA

Should you or a loved one be hit with these debilitating symptoms, nature may well help you with relief, to improve the symptoms.

FOODS/REMEDIES/LIFESTYLE ADJUSTMENTS – SCIENTIFICALLY VALIDATED

Foods

According to research at the
- *University of Medicine*
  &
- *University Hospital Center 'Mother Theresa'*
  (both in Albania's capital Tirana)

Mediterranean diet may be especially supportive in terms of GER/D relief.

With special reference to
-    fruits & vegetables
-    whole grains
  &
-    unsaturated fats

In more detail:

- ***Fruits***

Besides of the fact that fruits are an excellent nutritious source of, inter alia, vitamin C as well as vital minerals like potassium and magnesium, and fiber, they also may fight acid reflux.

This is especially true for, inter alia,
- apples
- pears
- melons
- berries
- avocados
- peaches
- bananas

- ***Vegetables***

With special reference to, inter alia,
- broccoli
- potatoes
- cauliflower
- spinach
- kale
- asparagus
- spinach
- green beans
- Brussel sprouts
- cucumbers

Being an excellent source of fiber as well, they are also low in sugar and 'wrong' types of fats like
- trans fats from processed foods
- saturated fats from meat/dairy
and therefore help to relieve acid reflux.

To be sure, however, this does not mean that fats are basically bad in terms of acid reflux. Rather, you may include healthy types of

- ***Fats***

in your diet to even support relief of acid reflux. As we find them, inter alia, in
- olive oil
- nuts & seeds
- avocado oil
- nut butter
- fatty fish

Also helpful are fiber-rich

- ***Whole grains***

like, inter alia,
- whole grain bread
- oatmeal
- brown rice

As scientifically verified also at the *Federal Research Center of Nutrition, Biotechnology and Food Safety* in Russia's capital Moscow.
Not to forget about lean

- ***Proteins***

as to be found in low-cholesterol diet such as, inter alia,
- chicken
- turkey
- fish
- beans
- lentils
- lean poultry
- seafood
- almonds

However, no frying please but baking/grilling/broiling or poaching instead.
Vice-versa, some other foods may be avoided such as, inter alia,
- calcium-rich foods (like milk/cheese) because of their content of saturated fats, such as
- meat with its usually high content of fatty acids and cholesterol
- too much salt

- trigger & flare-up foods, such as coffee/chocolate/mint/acidic
  drinks like orange juice & acidic foods like tomato sauce
which are counterproductive in terms of GER/D.

According to research at, inter alia,
- *University of Pennsylvania Perelman School of Medicine* in
  Philadelphia, PA
- *Weill Cornell Medical Center* in New York
- *Vrije Universiteit Brussel* in Brussels, Belgium
  as well as in Italy at
- *University of Milan* in Milan
- *University of Insubria* in Varese
- *University of Bari* in Bari
  &
- *University of 'Magna Graecia' of Catanzaro* in Catanzaro

Remedies

Additionally to appropriate GER/D relieving food you may also consider

- *slippery elm bark*

as a natural remedy which may not only soothe and coat stomach and
throat but relieves acid damage of the stomach by secreting mucus.

Based on research at, inter alia, *Stanford University* in Palo Alto, CA

Lifestyle adjustments

According to the U.S. *National Institute of Diabetes and Digestive and
Kidney Diseases,* lifestyle adjustments such as
- raising head during sleep
- managing body weight
- quit smoking
- staying hydrated
- no big meals at least 3 hours before bed
- avoiding carbonated drinks
may well contribute to GER/D relief as well.

IN A NUTSHELL

Heartburn with pain in the upper abdomen (i.e., acid reflux – also known by the abbreviation GER/D) is affecting some 20% of our adults. With special reference to certain unhealthy nutrition. Fortunately, nature is offering us specific foods, remedies and lifestyle adjustments to relieve this debilitating condition. As you have learned in this chapter.

21. PURPLE UP YOUR HEALTH

THE PHILOSOPHY BEHIND

As you know from our publications and beyond, your health depends on 2 basic pillars: healthy food and physical exercise. When talking about food, it's certainly nutritious components like vitamins and minerals, etc.

Not only. Since all fruits and vegetables are colored, this feature is of physiological and psychological relevance as well. With respect to one color specifically: purple. According to the U.S. *National Institutes of Health (NIH)*.

BENEFITS OF PURPLE FOOD – SCIENTIFICALLY VALIDATED

The specific benefit of purple-colored fruits and vegetables comes from its content of antioxidants (*anthocyanins*), i.e. plant pigments creating naturally blue and red colors in specific plants. With the capability of preventing and also repairing the damage of certain cells in our body.

In medical terms, this may help our body, inter alia, to avoid heart disease, fight cancer and, containing also antioxidants such as polyphenols, they may also cut down neurological conditions, including stress.

Let us briefly focus now on a sample of those purple-colored fruits and vegetables in favor of our health:

Fruits

- **Blueberries**

Rich in polyphenols like phenolic acids and flavonoids, blueberries may

-    alleviate inflammation
  &
-    boost our mood

- **Blackberries**

Rounded up with their contents of vitamins A/C/K and fiber, they may
-    reduce inflammation
  &
-    support mental capability

- **Purple grapes**

They may help to
- fight cancer
- support cardiovascular/arterial health
  &
- cut cholesterol

- **Concord grape juice**

May be well effective for
- spatial memory/memory function/reaction time
  &
- enhance calmness

- **Blackcurrants**

As they have high content of anthocyanins, they
- balance cholesterol level
  &
- support vision

- **Acai berries**

As research says, this purple-colored fruit may well support
- cognitive capacity
- cholesterol balancing
  &
- heart health

- **Plums**

Their antioxidants
- reduce inflammation
- support bone health
- improve digestion
- lower blood pressure
- cut doown blood sugar

- **Figs**

They may
- prevent cancer
  & support
- respiration
- digestion

- weight loss
- decrease of inflammation
- reproductive health

Vegetables

Similar benefits for our health we find in purple-colored vegetables like...

- **Eggplants**

Based on their rich content of phytochemicals and antioxidants such as, inter alia, flavonoids, ascorbic acid and phenolics, they may improve respiratory problems like
- asthma
  &
- bronchitis
as well as
- prevent liver damage

- **Purple corn**

This may well help to
- avoid certain cancers
  &
- diabetes
as well as
- cut down inflammation
  &
- body weight
and also
- support vision

- **Beetroots**

They may well
- prevent cancer
- lower blood pressure
- support heart health
- cut down inflammation
- improve digestion
- support gut health

- **Purple potatoes**

To cut down risk of
-    of colon cancer
     &
-    inflammation

- **Purple sweet potatoes**

Their health benefit of
-    strengthening our immunity
     and
-    cutting down inflammation
comes from their high anthocyanin power.

- **Purple carrots**

With special reference to their high amount of phytonutrients like anthocyanins as well as of alpha and beta anthocyanin, they also
-    strengthen immunity
     &
-    support our vision

- **Red cabbage**

Also this purple-colored vegetable may
-    fight cancer
     &
-    cardiovascular disease

Based on international research at, inter alia...

-    *Pennsylvania State University* in State Park, PA
-    *University of Western States* in Portland, OR
-    *Institute for Functional Medicine* in Federal Way, WA
-    *Cyprus University of Technology* in Lemesos, Cyprus
-    *University of Naples Federico II* in Portici, Italy
-    *University of Thessaly* in Magnisia, Greece
-    *Canakkale Onsekiz Mart University* in Canakkale, Turkey
-    *University of Guelph* in Guelph, Canada
-    *Luliu Hatiegano University of Medicine and Pharmacy*
     &
-    *University of Agricultural Sciences and Veterinary Medicine* (both in Cluj-Napoca, Romania)

IN A NUTSHELL

As indicated in our previous chapters and other publications, our health depends – besides (aerobic) physical exercise - on healthy diet. With its content of specific nutrients. More than that: also the color of our plant food plays a decisive role for our health – with special reference to *purple.*

22. STRAWBERRIES: MAGIC FRUIT FOR HEALTH?

THE PHILOSOPHY BEHIND

As you know from our blogs and other publications, fruits and vegetables are vital part of our health and longevity. In different ways, depending on the respective live-saving components involved, such as vitamins, minerals, and many others.

Still, there are many differences in this plant family in terms of respective natural constituents, and health benefits, accordingly.

Just let's have a look at our popular strawberries.

Although this may not be the time of the year for (fresh!) strawberries (grown without pesticides) but better you learn ahead of time (and mark your calendar) instead of being too late (which your body may not tolerate).

BENEFITS OF STRAWBERRIES – SCIENTIFICALLY VERIFIED

In fact, strawberries contain quite a few healthy compounds, like

- vitamins A/B-9 (folate)/C
- minerals magnesium/calcium/potassium/iron
- fiber
- protein

as well as other live-saving constituents with anti-inflammatory and antioxidant features. Such as certain

- flavonoids like quercetin/catechin/anthocyanins/kaempferol

according to the U.S. Department of Agriculture.

While, in fact, there are quite some health benefits involved in – fresh - strawberries (and also other berries), let' focus on those 3 of special reference in our modern/industrialized society.

A special benefit of these strawberries (and other berries) natural compounds is to prevent

Cancer

With special reference to types of

- breast/liver/prostate/lung/pancreatic/gastrointestinal/esophageal

cancer.

Based on research at, inter alia,
- *University of Maine* in Orono, ME
  &
- *Istanbul Yeni Yuzyil University* in Istanbul, Turkey

Another benefit lies with

Cardiovascular Disease

Based on research at, inter alia,
- *American University of Beirut*
  &
- *Lebanese International University*
  (both in Beirut, Lebanon)
  as well as
- *Alexandria University* in Alexandria, Egypt

Flavonoids like *anthocyanins* of strawberries may lower the risk of

- **Heart attack**

Also, *quercetin* may reduce the risk of

- **Atherosclerosis**

According to research at *Tezpur University* in Napaam, India.

Both supported by *potassium* in strawberries, according to the U.S. *Centers for Disease Control and Prevention (CDC)*.

More than that. Based on research at, inter alia, the *Second Affiliated Hospital of Nanchang University* in Nanchang, China, these flavonoids may also cut the risk of

- **Stroke**

Another health benefit of strawberries comes with its content of *potassium*, in terms of

- **High Blood Pressure**

by counterbalancing the unhealthy effects of sodium.

According to, inter alia, the *University Hospital Lausanne* in Lausanne, Switzerland.

IN A NUTSHELL

Although it's not yet the time to buy – fresh – strawberries (& grown without pesticides!), you better learn ahead about their health benefits involved. With special reference to cancer and cardiovascular disease – the most debilitating health concerns of our modern/industrialized society.

23. SAVE YOUR HEALTH FROM HYPOMAGNESEMIA

THE PHILOSOPHY BEHIND

Our health and longevity is highly dependent on natural nutrients, with special reference to minerals. Just as 2-time Nobel Prize laureate Professor Linus Pauling from *Oregon State University* has stated a historic medical principle: *"You can trace every sickness, every disease and every ailment to a mineral deficiency."*

Especially a deficiency of *magnesium* - medical term: *hypomagnesemia*. As verified by conventional medicine inter alia at *Sapienza University of Rome* in Italy's capital Rome.

E.g., in terms of cardiovascular disease. Just to indicate the proverbial medical tip of the iceberg as the most debilitating disease of our time (followed by cancer and diabetes). With special reference to
- heart disease
- high blood pressure/hypertension
- stroke

Besides many other health issues caused by magnesium deficiency – of which more than 50% citizens of our 'modern' society are affected. I.e. with less than 0.75 millimoles per liter (mmol/l) of magnesium in the blood.

Including
- blood sugar (diabetes)
- cognitive capability
- migraine headache
- kidney disease
  and not to forget about
- impact on, yes, *longevity*.
  &
- health of muscles.
  In fact, **magnesium** is almost indispensable for well-functioning muscle contractions.

As verified scientifically at, inter alia,
- *Harvard School of Public Health* in Boston, MA
- *University of Hertfordshire* in Hartfield, UK

- *University of Palermo* in Palermo, Italy
- *University of Western Australia* in Perth, Australia

Finally not to forget about the impact of magnesium on our – yes - *longevity.*

Supported by research, inter alia, in California at the *University of California in Berkeley* & *Children's Hospital Oakland Research Institute* in Oakland.

Symptoms

In fact, hypomagnesemia is realized manifoldly early prior to harsh effect by respective symptoms such as, inter alia,
- exhaustion/weakness
- tremors
- myoclonic twitches (face & other parts of body)
- nausea/vomiting
- twitches
- change of personality

as magnesium is related to more than 300 (!) enzyme reactions, according to U.S. *National Institutes o Health (NIH).*

NATURE'S ANSWER

Fortunately, nature is giving us plenty of (non-processed) foods with magnesium content we may well appreciate to avoid hypomagnesemia by incorporating those in our menu.

According to the U.S. *National Institutes of Health (NIH)*, this includes - inter alia -

- whole wheat bread
- spinach
- rice
- potatoes
- black/kidney beans
- yogurt
- edamer
- fortified cereals
- avocados
- apples
- bananas
- raisins

- oatmeal
- fish (like salmon & halibut)
- nuts (primarily peanuts/almonds/cashews)
- broccoli
- carrots
- peanut butter
- chicken breast
- milk

IN A NUTSHELL

Healthy diet is a basic prerequisite for our health and longevity. With special reference to vitamins and minerals – magnesium just as one priority. In this chapter you learned about the consequences of magnesium deficiency – *hypomagnesemia* – and how to overcome it, naturally.

24. FAST FOOD: GOOD OR BAD FOR YOUR HEALTH?

THE PHILOSOPHY BEHIND

We certainly can't live without nutrition. However, our modern society tries to spend least time for it, in favor of other timely responsibilities. Without giving much thought to its quality. As long as we consume the appropriate amount of calories - ? Neglecting the fact that our health and longevity is not only a matter of calories but got to be based on certain nutrients.

In many cases this type of 'fast' food is not only short of vital nutrients like certain antioxidants, fiber, etc., but loaded with unhealthy ingredients. Such as salt, sugar, saturated fat, trans fats, processed preservatives and high amount of calories – just to indicate the proverbial tip of the iceberg.

According to international medical research at, inter alia, *Shahid Beheshti University of Medical Sciences* in Iran's capital Tehran.

Unfortunately yet, the majority of our population is consuming too much of these unhealthy food components. According to the U.S. Department of Health and Human Service & the U.S. Department of Agriculture.

MEDICAL CONSEQUENCES – SCIENTIFICALLY VERIFIED

In fact, this unhealthy nutritional part of our diet has serious short- & long-term effects for our health – besides overweight/obesity - as follows (just to indicate some of the most important ones).

- ### *Heart disease*

An overconsumption of salt has well an impact on blood pressure. With the potential consequence of stroke and heart attack.

I.e., the high level of salt we usually find in fast food has a negative impact on the blood vessels – and blood pressure, accordingly.

According to international research at, inter alia, the
- *University of Illinois at Chicago* in Chicago, IL
  &
- *Josip Juraj Strossmayer University of Osijek* in Osijek, Croatia

Also, the usually high amount of trans fats in fast food has well a negative effect on cholesterol, as it raises 'bad' cholesterol (LDL) and cuts down 'good' cholesterol (HDL). Complicating heart disease even more.

- ***Blood sugar irregularity***

Added sugar and refined carbohydrates in fast food lets blood sugar soar up to the region of diabetes. Also causing an unusual high surge of insulin, dropping blood sugar with giving us the feeling of tiredness.

Based on research at, inter alia,
- *Northern Arizona University* in Flagstaff, AZ
  &
- *Nutritional Research Foundation* in Flemington, NJ.

- ***Inflammation***

As you may know from our previous blogs and publications, inflammation stands behind each kind of disease.

Unfortunately, the high amount of saturated fat we find usually in fast food, worsens this inflammation even more.

Based on research at, inter alia, *Shahid Beheshti University of Medical Sciences* in Tehran, Iran.

Along with higher degree of inflammation, this type of fast food may offer less protection for autoinflammatory diseases, infections, cancer, and allergies, etc.

According to research at, inter alia, the *University of Bonn* in Bonn, Germany.

The lack of fiber in most cases of fast food is also responsible for

- ***Digestive irregularities***

such as diverticular disease, constipation and of cutting down healthy gut bacteria.

Based on research at, inter alia, the *University of Washington School of Medicine* in Seattle, WA.

In this context, we have also to see the fact that fast food is responsible for

- ***Overweight/obesity***

as a consequence of its high amount of calories. According to the U.S. Department of Agriculture.

Leading to different health issues, as confirmed by the U.S. Centers for Disease Control and Prevention (CDC).

- ***Allergies***

The unfavorable nutritional criteria of fast food may also be responsible for asthma, eczema and rhinoconjunctivitis.

According to research at, inter alia,
- *University of Newcastle* in New Lambton, Australia
  &
- *Sichuan University* in Chengdu, China

- ***Lower memory capacity***

The risk of Alzheimer's disease and Parkinson's disease may well be caused, inter alia, by saturated fat and simple carbohydrates in fast food.

Based on international research at, inter alia,
- *State University of New Jersey* in New Brunswick, NJ
- *Federal University of Rio Grande do Sul* in Porto Alegre, Brazil
  &
- *University of New South Wales* in Kensington, Australia

Not to forget that the unhealthy implications of fast foods may well responsible also for some

- ***Mental impact***

like anxiety and depression.

According to *Binghamton University* in Binghamton, NY.

IN A NUTSHELL

With so called 'fast food' we may well save time for other responsibilities in our daily life. Unfortunately, not our health in physical and mental terms. Because of the manifold unfavorable ingredients of this type of food. Indicated by a sample of related health issues (as the proverbial 'tip of the iceberg').

25. BREAST PAIN – BREAST CANCER?

THE PHILOSOPHY BEHIND

Two thirds of females are affected by breast pain at least once in their life. Primarily in their so called 'child-bearing age' between 15 and 40, the so called reproductive years.

On the other hand, *breast cancer* is not only one of the most debilitating diseases for women, it is in fact the most diagnosed type of cancer in women worldwide.

Leaves us with the question, if breast pain (medical term *mastalgia)* is the one and only symptom of breast cancer at all.

POTENTIAL CAUSE OF BREAST PAIN – SCIENTIFICALLY VERIFIED

In fact, there are quite a few conditions related to breast pain. To avoid unnecessary panicking in cases of breast pain, let's rationalize the situation in following.

Starting with the least 'dramatic' cause of breast pain:

- *Unfavorable bra fit*

This can happen in cases where, e.g.,
- a bra is too tight
  or
- where it is incorporating a wire hurting the breast tissue or just the skin

In cases like these, it may be helpful to wear a supportive and more comfortable bra especially in situations when exercising.

This helped at least two thirds of females when exercising, according to research by
- *MVR Cancer Center & Research Institute* in Kerala, India
  &
- *Service Institute of Medical Sciences* in Lahore, Pakistan

- ***Mastitis***

Inflammation of breast tissue (medical term *mastitis)* and swelling of the breast according to infection may be another problem. As the result of breast feeding or otherwise, potentially causing breast pain as well.

With following additional potential symptoms:

- fever
- headaches
- warmth in parts of the breast
- flu-like feelings

According to the *American Cancer Society*.

Also

- ***Medications***

may potentially cause breast pain as well. Like ones for
- treating cardiovascular problems with respect to irregular heart rhythm/congestive heart failure/high blood pressure, etc.
- potassium-sparing diuretics
- mental health conditions

According to the U.S. *National Breast Cancer Foundation* in Dallas, TX.

- ***Hormonal changes***

Regularly, there are hormonal changes before periods start. These may well cause swollen/tender breasts with pain (termed 'cyclic breast pain').

Potentially related to additional symptoms before the period starts, according to the *Office on Women's Health* at the *U.S. Department of Health and Human Services* in Washington, D.C.

These symptoms ('premenstrual syndromes' - PMS) may be, inter alia,
- tiredness
- mood swings
- constipation/diarrhea
- headaches
- bloating
- acne
- poor sleep

While PMS is usually temporary only, to wear a supportive/comfortable bra also in this case is recommended.

However, this kind of breast pain and related symptoms may also occur as the result of other hormonal changes, like those during the time of pregnancy as well as the beginning of menopause.

These hormonal fluctuations can also cause a type of relatively harmless but potentially painful situation.

- ***Fibrocystic breast disease***

is giving the breast a lumpy feeling.

With symptoms such as, inter alia,
- sensitive nipples
- itchiness
- tenderness

Especially before period starts but mainly stops after menopause.

According to research at, inter alia,
- *University of Michigan* in Ann Artbor, Michigan
- *University of Pretoria* in Pretoria, South Africa
  &
- *Agha Khan University* in Karachi, Pakistan

- ***Neck-back-shoulder injuries/sprains***

Another reason for breast pain may be a pinched nerve root due to inflammation or damage in the neck/back/shoulder caused by injury or sprain and this pain could well be felt also in the breast.

According to research at, inter alia, *Mugla Sitki Kocman University* in Mugla, Turkey.

- ***Chest wall pain***

can happen as well.

As a type of pain in the chest, giving the feeling of being located in the breast.

With symptoms such as, inter alia,
- sharp/burning pain
  &
- pain worsening in cases of movements

As the actual result of, inter alia,
- gallstones
- rheumatoid arthritis
- angina
  etc.

Based on research at the organization *Breast Cancer Now* in London, UK.

- ***Breast cysts***

Known as fluid-filled sacs, they are happening frequently in situations of pre menopause. Not necessarily but potentially felt as painful.

According to the **Stockport NHS Foundation Trust** in Stockport, UK.

Finally – yes –

- ***Breast cancer***

may also well be one of the causes behind of breast pain.

As verified by the U.S. *Centers for Disease Control and Prevention (CDC)*.

Related to symptoms, such as, inter alia,
- swelling/thickening in parts of breast
- breast change (size/shape)
- red inflamed/flaky skin around nipple or other part
- lump in breast

Not only this.

According to the *American Cancer Society,* conventional breast cancer therapy with surgery and radiation can lead to scar tissue and well cause, inter alia,
- change the appearance of the breast (make it firmer/rounder)
- pain/numbness when scar tissue is around nerves
- a lump to be formed if scar is around stitch from surgery

IN A NUTSHELL

Two thirds of females are affected by breast pain at least once in their life.
On the other hand, breast cancer is in fact the most diagnosed type
of cancer in women worldwide. In this chapter we clarify the link between
both.

26. SAVE YOUR HEART & HEALTH WITH SUNSHINE?

THE PHILOSOPHY BEHIND

Spending most per capita for conventional medicine in the industrialized world, the U.S. is foremost in this field of expertise. With special reference to our cardiovascular system.

Historically documented by, inter alia,
- 1st open heart surgery worldwide (Dr. Michael E. DeBakey)
- 1st modern cardiologist worldwide (Dr. Paul Dudley White – personal physician of U.S. president Dwight Eisenhower)
- 1st artificial heart transplant worldwide (Dr. Denton Cooley)
- 1st heart repair with stem cells worldwide (Dr. Ed Marban)

The back side of this shiny medal:

According to statistics of the *World Health Organization (WHO)*, in our industrialized world (with the U.S. on top),
- 86% of non-age-related deaths
  &
- 77% of all ailments combined

are the consequence of 'chronic' diseases – unsolved with conventional medicine.

With
- heart failure
  on top, followed by
- cancer
  (half a century after U.S. President Nixon declared the 'War on Cancer')
  &
- diabetes (with a most prescribed drug worldwide, being rich of side effects -but offering no cure)

In fact, according to *WHO*, almost 20 million people die each year of heart disease worldwide. I.e. one third of all (premature) deaths are cardiovascular related. According to the U.S. *Centers for Disease Control and Prevention (CDC)*.

A vicious cycle? Not necessarily...

NATURE'S POWER OF SUNSHINE – SCIENTIFICALLY VERIFIED

As you know from our previous publications, nature offers us many (not to say: unlimited...) remedies and modalities to bolster our health and longevity. With special reference to minerals and vitamins.

Including vitamin D. Not only to support bones and teeth but our immune system in general.

Now we learn from research of the *Australian Centre for Precision Health* at the *University of South Australia* in Adelaide that a lack of vitamin D in our body may have quite a negative impact on our heart health specifically.

As verified, inter alia, also by the *Providence Saint John's Health Center* in Santa Monica, CA.

Leaves us with the question how and where to get vitamin D for our body.

According to, inter alia, the *University of Florida* in Gainesville, FL, there are foods containing vitamin D such as:
- cooked sockeye salmon
- drained canned tuna/sardines
- fortified milk
- fortified breakfast cereal
- hard boiled eggs
- low fat vanilla yogurt
- fortified orange juice

Even more, exposure to the sun is another way to tap vitamin D and store it in our body. With the ultimate benefit to receive adequate vitamin D naturally as our skin produces vitamin D when exposed to UVB rays of the sun in a moderate way. But be aware of the UV index: if its higher than 1, you should use sun protection and caution.

According to research at, inter alia, the *University of Bonn* and the *Heart and Diabetes Center North Rhine-Westphalia* in Bad Oyenhausen – both in Germany.

With basic factors involved:

- How much skin exposed?
  Basically, any exposure of our skin to sunlight produces vitamin D. However, the more skin you expose (e.g., additionally to face and hands), the more vitamin D it will produce.

- How long stay exposed?
  According to the *U.S. Vitamin D Council* in San Luis Obispo, Ca, stay exposed for moderate time (20 *Minutes)* in areas and at times with an UV index of 1 or less seems appropriate. This is usually the case in the morning or before sunset, even in areas with high UV index during the day.
- Sun exposure got to be 'natural', i.e. not through a window which blocks UVB rays.

Unfortunately yet, long office hours and spending much time in front of TV, thus diminishing sun exposure, may well be counterproductive especially for heart health.

IN A NUTSHELL

For our health in general, and our cardiovascular system specifically, natural support with certain vitamins is indispensable. With special reference to vitamin D. While we can – and should - take this vitamin, besides many other healthy nutrients, from appropriate food, nature offers us also the sun as a prime source - with caution and moderation. For free!

27. SAVE YOUR MENTAL HEALTH NATURALLY

THE PHILOSOPHY BEHIND

As you know from our medical blogs, books & seminars, good **health** depends on 2 basic factors: healthy diet & (aerobic) exercise. Physically & mentally. Our mental power is just the other side of the shiny medal.

With reference to potential mental disorders like, e.g., anxiety, depression and post-traumatic stress disorder (PTSD) – the latter also a manifold veteran-related health issue.

Appreciating the fact that more than 20% of our adult population nationally is hit by mental problems.

Covid-19 pandemic impact

This may have special priority in our time of the Covid-19 pandemic.

According to a recent international study, elaborated at the *University of Queensland* in Brisbane, Australia, the current Corona pandemic has added
-     53 million cases of major depression disorder
      &
-     76 million of anxiety disorder
  worldwide.

This is in line with findings in Canada at the *University of Ottawa Department of Family Medicine & Ottawa Hospital,* according to which outpatient healthcare visits for mental health soared because of this pandemic.

Fortunately, there are sometimes less common therapies for your mental support you may not want to miss.

NATURAL SUPPORT FOR MENTAL HEALTH – SCIENTIFICALLY VERIFIED

Just let's pick 2 remedies and 2 modalities for easy self-administration.

Starting with the nutritional remedy

Omega-3 polyunsaturated fatty acids

Recommended by *Mental Health America (MHA),* a leading non-profit organization in the field of mental illness. Located in Alexandria, Virginia.

To support not only our mental well-being but also support the health of our heart.

With special reference to, inter alia, following mental health problems:

- cognitive impairment
- bipolar disorder
- depression (including seasonal affective disorders/SAD as a major depression)
- attention deficit hyperactivity disorder (ADHD)
- schizophrenia

Another powerful natural remedy is the plant

Kava Kava

(also briefly known as 'kava') grown on the islands of the Western Pacific region and used by the folks since centuries, becoming popular all over the U.S. meanwhile.

With special reference to mild/moderate anxiety, stress and inflammation.

According to research at, inter alia, the *University of North Carolina* in Chapel Hill, NC.

Now to the 'modalities';

Animal partnership

Roughly two thirds of American households share their premises with a pet. For most of those, pets - especially cats and dogs – not only are "man's best friend" but the best friends and companions at all. With the overriding benefit of being happy most of the time together and support relaxation.

Not only this. Most of us are not aware that these pets are helping us to feel well and even more: they help us to stay – or become – healthy.

In fact, folks with a lovely cat or dog tested much less positive for stress, anxiety, impulsiveness and depression.

Scientifically validated, inter alia, at
- *University of Florida* in Gainesville, Florida
- *University of Torino* in Torino, Italy
  &
- *National Alliance on Mental Illness (NAMI)* in Arlington, Virginia

Finally, we may briefly focus on

Yoga

Native to India since thousands of years, yoga (derived from Sanskrit word 'Yuj' – meaning 'to join') is meanwhile established also in our culture. For addressing – and connecting - our physical, mental and spiritual well-being.

With quite a few physical and mental health benefits such as, inter alia,
- stress reduction
- better balance
- strengthening of the immunity
- weight management

In terms of our mental capacity, with special reference to disorders like, inter alia,
- depression
- attention deficit hyperactivity disorder (ADHD)
- post-traumatic stress disorder (PTSD)
- schizophrenia

According to, inter alia, the *Aslang Ayurveda Hospital and Research Centre* in Kathmandu, Nepal.

Offering us an overall increased quality of life.

IN A NUTSHELL

To save our health – physically & mentally - depends on 2 basic factors: healthy diet & (aerobic) exercise. Fortunately, nature offers us additional remedies and modalities for our mental support, as indicated in this scientifically verified elaboration.

28. SUPPORT SEX LIFE FOR YOUR HEALTH?

THE PHILOSOPHY BEHIND

When 'sex' comes to the mind, most of us may think/talk about off the record, as this subject may seem somehow *indecent*. At best, we talk and feel that somebody *else* may have *sex appeal*.

However, we may not want to overlook that our world's population of more than 7 billion is a direct result of – yes – our ancestor's *sex* activity. You yourself – and me – included.

More than that.

BENEFIT OF SEX FOR OUR HEALTH

According to recent/conventional medical science, sex activity is related to our health – in a positive way.

With special reference to those 2 health issues topping the statistics of the World Health Organization (WHO) about chronic diseases with non-age related premature deaths in our industrialized world: heart disease, followed by cancer.

According to latest research at the *University of Washington* in Seattle, WA, cancer diagnoses have risen dramatically worldwide from 18.7 million in 2010 to 23.6 million today. With cancer deaths soaring from 8.29 million to 10 million same time. Half a century after U.S. president Nixon had declared the 'War on Cancer' in 1971.

Ranking the U.S. only #31 in the WHO statistics of global life expectancy. Despite of spending most for medicine in the industrialized world: $10,000 per capita annually.

Just let's focus on research at the *Institute of Brain, Behaviour and Mental Health* at the *University of Manchester* in Manchester & Salford, UK.

According to their scientific findings, the risk of *heart disease* may well decrease by 50% if having sex at least 2 times a week. In comparison to folks having sex just one time a month.

In terms of cancer:

Men practicing sex 4 times a week may lower their risk of developing prostate cancer by 30% unlike those with sex only 2 times the week.

Based on research at *Johns Hopkins University/Bloomberg School of Public Health* in Baltimore, MD.

NATURAL SUPPORT WITH HERBS – SCIENTIFICALLY VALIDATED

In order to support sex life naturally by itself and overcome erectile dysfunction specifically, medical science recommends at least 2 specific herbs, as follows.

Muira puama

As an extract from a bush native to Brazil, it may well improve the situation of erectile dysfunction, according to research at *Vendome Hospital* in Vendome, France.

This is in line with scientific findings at *Ottawa Hospital Research Institute* in Ottawa, Canada.

According to these findings, this herb enhanced sexual desire in men by 60% and women by 65%, improved also erectile dysfunction by 50% in males.

With reference to a daily value of 100 mg muira puama extract.

Fenugreek

This herb native in the Mediterranean as a sex booster by increasing levels of testosterone, according to research at *University of Queensland School of Medicine* in Brisbane, Australia.

The *Aman Hospital and Research Center* in Vadodara, India, confirmed this scientific finding. Based on a study confirming enhancement of female libido in almost half of prospects with daily value of 500 mg fenugreek for 42 days.

IN A NUTSHELL

Although thought & talked about usually off the record, as a seemingly indecent issue, sex life may well support our health. With special reference to heart disease and cancer. As scientifically validated in this elaboration.

29. SAVE HEALTH WITH BERRIES FROM WW II?

THE PHILOSOPHY BEHIND

As you know latest from our publications and seminars: healthy diet plays a central role for our physical and mental well-being and existence. With special reference to certain nutrients our body needs to survive.

In this respect, the best 'fountain of youth' for vital nutrients is certainly nature's kingdom of edible plants. With special reference to certain vegetables and fruits, each of those incorporating not only one specific nutrient but a whole complexity. In terms of vitamins, minerals and beyond. In most cases, to help with different contemporary health issues each.

While we all know, e.g., the proverb that 'an apple a day keeps the doctor away', there are additionally highly valuable fruits we may not want to miss for our good health.

Like *bilberries*. The round and purple-colored European cousins of our North American blueberries. With its name 'bilberry' coming from Danish 'bollebar' which means *dark berry*.

In fact, bilberry is high in natural chemical *anthocyanins* (i.e. vital anti-inflammatory antioxidants). Additionally, they are an excellent source of powerful nutrients such as vitamin C, catechins and quercetin.

According to research at, inter alia, *Hong Kong Polytechnic University* in Hong Kong.

According to the U.S. governmental *National Institutes of Health (NIH)*, this fruit supported health already in the Middle Ages with respect to, inter alia,
- inflammation
- diarrhea
- urinary problems

just to pick a sample.

And during WW II, British pilots of fighter jets consumed bilberry for potentially better vision during night.

With the benefit for eye health by reducing, inter alia,

- pain
- fatigue
- heaviness
- uncomfortable sensation
  and
- foreign body sensation

as verified by research at *Keio University School of Medicine* in Japan's capital Tokyo.

But can bilberries be helpful also in terms of debilitating health issues of today?

HEALTH BENEFITS OF BILBERRY – SCIENTIFICALLY VALIDATED

Basically, this fruit may well have a positive effect on

- **inflammation**

which, to be sure, stands behind each disease.

Based on research, inter alia, in Malaysia at
- *Universiti Kebangsaan Malaysia* in Kuala Lumpur
  &
- *Universiti Putra Malaysia* in Selangor Darul Ehsan

Even more. According to
- *University of North Carolina* in Chapel Hill, NC
  as well as in Florida at the
- *University of Miami Miller School of Medicine* in Miami
  &
- *Mount Sinai Medical Center* at Miami Beach

bilberry may also help with cardiovascular risk factors.

E.g., by

- **lowering high blood pressure**

according to research at the *University of Oslo* in Norway's capital Oslo.

Inter alia, because of bilberries' high content of polyphenols. As verified by the U.S. *National Institutes of Health (NIH)*.

Also, bilberries may

- ***lower LDL cholesterol***

based on research at *Pusan National University* in Busan, South Korea. (Please note: the different spelling of Pusan/Busan is official.)

Additionally, it may help with management of blood sugar in cases of

- ***Diabetes 2***

including to increase insulin secretion.

According to research at, inter alia,
- *Danube University of Krems* in Krems, Austria
- *University of Bologna* in Bologna, Italy
- *University of Aberdeen* in Aberdeen UK
- *King Abdulaziz University* in Jeddah, Saudi Arabia
  as well as
- *University of Eastern Finland*
  &
- *Kuopio University Hospital*
  (both in Kuopio, Finland)

IN A NUTSHELL

To become and stay healthy, certain edible plants play a vital role. Like bilberry. This fruit is not only important for our well-being and health in general but especially for debilitating diseases of our time. Because of its complex nutritional content. To make sure you get hold of all the nutrients and not just an extract, preferably consume the whole fruit, fresh or dried.

30. DIABETICS: ENJOY LIFE WITH TASTY FOOD!

THE PHILOSOPHY BEHIND

As you know latest from my previous publications, the US. Is foremost in conventional medicine of the industrialized world.

Despite of that, 86% of non-age-related (premature) deaths and 77% of all ailments in general, are the consequence of *chronic* (unsolved) diseases. According to the *World Health Organization (WHO)* and verified by the US. Governmental *Centers for Disease Control and Prevention (CDC).* With heart failure and cancer on top, followed by diabetes.

With special reference to the fact that the most prescribed drug for diabetes worldwide (with a turnover of more than 100 billion dollars) got 69 side effects but no cure.

The only way out of this vicious cycle is what U.S. Navy has declared as its new mission also for our veterans: Alternative Medicine. With healthy diet in the forefront.

FOODS FOR DIABETICS – SCIENTIFICALLY VERIFIED

According to US. governmental *National Institute of Diabetes and Digestive and Kidney Disease*, scientifically proven at, inter alia, the *University of Leeds* in Leeds, UK,

Vegetables

...are basically important for diabetics because of their high content of vitamins, minerals, fiber, protein. As these basic nutrients are keeping blood sugar in balance.

With special reference to, inter alia,
- Goreens
- broccoli
- tomatoes
- carrots
- Potatoes
- green peas

- corn
- peppers

Based on research, inter alia, in the UK at
- *King's College*
- *Queen Mary's University*
  (both London)
- *University of Liverpool* in Liverpool
- *University of Aberdeen* in Aberdeen

Beans

are also an excellent source for proteins and fiber, helping to digest fewer carbohydrates.

Especially following members of the bean family:
- black beans
- kidney beans
- pinto beans
- white beans
- garbanzo beans

Verified by research at, inter alia, *Zhejiang University* in Zhejiang, China.

Proteins

Since protein is very important for diabetics, increasing blood sugar only moderate, they may well consider consuming, inter alia, following sources of protein, according to research at, inter alia, *Andrews University* in Berrien Springs, MI.

Plant-based sources

- lentils
- pinto beans
- black beans
- falafel
- kidney beans
- peas
- tempeh
- hummus
- edamame
- tofu

<u>*Animal-based sources*</u>

- fish
  such as, inter alia,
    - salmon
    - tuna
    - white fish
    - sardines
- eggs
- skinless turkey breast
- boneless chicken breast/strips

These plant- and animal-related proteins are scientifically recommended also by, inter alia, *Sheffield Hallam University* in Sheffield, UK.

Not to overlook the fact that

Fruits

are basically helpful for diabetics as well.

Although they do contain sugar, this type of sugar does not harm the diabetic.

What really counts in favor of the diabetic, is the *low glycemic index (GI)* of whole fruits like, inter alia

- apples
- pears
- cherries
- avocados
- blackberries
- grapefruit
- strawberries
- plums

As scientifically verified at, inter alia,
- *University of Oxford* in Oxford, UK
  &
- *Peking University Health Sciences Center* in China's capital Beijing

Whole grains

are a beneficial part of nutrition for diabetics as well, as they are balancing out the glycemic index (GI).

With special reference to, inter alia,
- whole grain bread
- whole wheat flour
- oatmeal
- barley
- millet
- cornmeal
- amaranth
- quinoa
- wild rice
- legume pasta

Scientifically supported also by *Diabetes UK* in London, UK.

Dairy

on the other hand, may be very positive with respect to insulin secretion.

According to *California Dairy Research Foundation* in Davis, CA.

As scientifically verified at, inter alia,
- *Harvard School of Public Health* in Boston, MA
  &
- *Lund University* in Lund, Sweden

With special reference to, inter alia, following types of dairy:

- cottage cheese
- parmesan
- ricotta
- low fat/skimmed milk/Greek or plain yogurt

For even more nutritional enjoyment, diabetics may add up these very healthy foods with certain

Desserts

Such as, inter alia,

- 100% fruit popsicles
- desserts with sugar-free gelatin

- pudding/ice cream with no or low calorie sweeteners like stevia/erythritol

Based on research, inter alia, in Spain's capital Madrid at the
- *Spanish Medical Research Centre in Diabetes and Associated Metabolic Disorders*
  &
- *Institute of Food Science and Technology and Nutrition*

And if you favor any

Snacks

between regular meal times, just choose diabetes-friendly ones like

- celery sticks
- carrots
- homemade popcorn

just to pick a small sample.

According to the *California Dairy Research Foundation n Davis, CA*

COUNTERPRODUCTIVE FOOD FOR DIABETICS

Leaves us with the question if and which types of food diabetics better cut down and out.

These are, according to the *Dietary Guidelines for Americans* of the governmental *U.S. Department of Agriculture (USDA)*, inter alia,

- packaged/fast foods
- sugar in candy/cakes/ice cream
- white bread/pasta/rice
- saturated/trans fats
- sugary drinks/cereals
- red/processed meat

IN A NUTSHELL

To manage diabetes requires quite some lifestyle adjustments. Fortunately yet, you can still enjoy life with a kingdom of tasty foods you don't have to cut out as a diabetic but rather incorporate in your daily diet. Instead of following a strict medical regimen nutritionally.

31. HOW RELIEVE PSORIASIS NATURALLY?

THE PHILOSOPHY BEHIND

According to *World Psoriasis Day* consortium, 8 million U.S. Citizens – and 125 million inhabitants of this planet – are struck with psoriasis. While many health issues may vanish with treatment, psoriasis is a 'chronic' autoimmune situation where the immune system is responsible for the overproduction of skin cells. Causing thick and red scaly patches (plaque). In most cases on scalp, knees and elbows. Itchy and painful.

Although not life-threatening, the situation is still inconvenient and therefore usually suppressed with medical synthetics from the shelve, without solving the problem. Rather, resulting in side effects and symptoms of additional health issues – going round in circles, accordingly.

To relieve this vicious cycle, nature gives us quite a few opportunities we may not want to overlook. To cut down respective symptoms and side effects.

Let us focus on an assortment of appropriate remedies/modalities to be applied on the skin and inside of our body.

NATURAL SUPPORT – SCIENTIFICALLY VERIFIED

To start with natural treatment on top of the skin, irradiation of

- ***Sunlight***

is certainly the most natural – and economic – way to expose to UVB rays in order to relieve the psoriatic issue. Without overstating time wise, to avoid sunburn.

According to the U.S. *National Psoriasis Foundation (NPF)*.

Also

- ***Tea tree oil***

a yellow essential oil derived from the leaves of the anti-inflammatory/antifungal/antibacterial/antiviral tea tree plant *Melaleuca Alternifolia* may well help to relieve *psoriasis*.

Native to Australia, where it has been used since a century for treating skin conditions the natural way.

According to the *University of Western Australia* in Crawley.

Another treatment of itchy psoriatic skin may well be an

- ***Oatmeal bath***

and

- ***Wet dressing***

Based on research at, inter alia, *Maulana Azad Medical College* in New Delhi, India.

Similar to using

- ***Wet wraps***

in this case, according to *Mayo Clinic* in Rochester, MN.

- ***Aloe vera***

is recommended to cut down inflammation and scaling of psoriasis according to research, inter alia, at the *University of Rome* in Italy's capital.

Applying

- ***Apple cider vinegar***

On the skin to soothe burning and itching of psoriatic skin is recommended by, inter alia, *Wayne State University School of Medicine* in Detroit, MI.

Because of its antioxidant and antimicrobial properties.

- ***Oregon grape***

(botanical term *mahonia aquifolium*) may cut down the immune response in cases of *psoriasis*.

According to *Memorial University of Newfoundland* in St. John's, Canada. verified also by *Loyola University Chicago* in Maywood, Il.

To shift natural treatment under skin, let's first take a look at

- ***Probiotics***

as it is found in yogurt and in fermented foods such as
- *Kombucha*
  (sweetened black tea)
- *Miso/tempeh*
  (soybean-based)
- *Kefir*
  (fermented dairy/similar to yogurt)

According to research at, inter alia,
- *University of Latvia* in Riga, Latvia
  &
- *University of Cambridge* in Cambridge, UK

- ***Curcumin***

as the active part in spice *turmeric* relieves inflammation of the skin and psoriasis in general.

Based on research at, inter alia, *University of Florence* in Florence, Italy.

And in China at
- *Peking University School and Hospital of Stomatology* in Beijing
  &
- *Xi'an Jiaotong University* in Xi'an

Also recommended is

- ***Capsaicin***

a component of red peppers, known as a fighter of inflammation by research at, inter alia, *Stony Brook University* in Stony Brook, NY.

IN A NUTSHELL

Psoriasis as a long-term ('chronic') skin disease with no cure by conventional medicine yet, can be relieved softly with natural remedies we have indicated as an assortment in this elaboration. Based on scientific evidence. For the convenience of those millions affected.

32. RELIEVE RHEUMATOID ARTHRITIS NATURALLY

THE PHILOSOPHY BEHIND

Rheumatoid arthritis (RA) is one of the debilitating and painful 'chronic' (speak: unsolved) health issues in our 'modern' times. Based on swelling and inflammation of our joints, loss of muscle mass, etc. causing pain all over the body. With special reference to the upper part such as hands/elbows/wrists/shoulders as well the lower part like feet/knees/ankles.

Leading to disability and reduced quality of life.

Usually treated by conventional medicine with synthetic drugs to suppress symptoms temporarily. With side effects. And by replacing knees and/or hips in some cases. Rounding up the vicious cycle.

For natural relief, the *American College of Rheumatology* in Atlanta, Georgia, recommends physical exercises in order to
- improve movement/daily function/sleep
  and above all
- manage/reduce pain

TYPES OF RA PHYSICAL EXERCISES – SCIENTIFICALLY VERIFIED

Just start with the easiest and still very helpful exercise – brisk

- ***Walking***

for at least 150 minutes per week. Starting slowly and increasing the speed.

As recommended by the U.S. governmental *Centers for Disease Control and Prevention (CDC)*.

- ***Stretching***

is another helpful exercise, in order to loosen stiffness for better movement of joints, knees, elbows and hands.

To practice daily for at least 20-30 seconds each stretch and repeating it 2-3 times.

After warming up ahead for 3-5 minutes by pumping arms while standing or sitting

According to international research at, inter alia,
- *University of Wolverhampton* in Wolverhampton, UK
  &
- *University of Thessaly* in Trikala, Greece

- ### *Cycling*

In both ways – stationary indoor and aerobic outdoor – may not only build endurance but also reduce stiffness and increase leg strength.

Based on research at, inter alia, *University of Wolverhampton* in Wolverhampton, UK.

- ### *Swimming*

and other water exercises, gently performed, is excellent as it relieves stress on joints and stiffness.

According to, inter alia, *Manchester Metropolitan University* in Manchester, UK.

- ### *Strength training*

To strengthen the muscles around joints – e.g. by resistance band – may also be helpful.

According to the U.S. *Centers for Disease Control and Prevention (CDC).*

To cross the cultural border -

- ### *Yoga & Tai Chi*

may be helpful as well with its breathing exercises, postures and flowing movements and meditation to relieve RA symptoms in terms of, inter alia,
- stress reduction
- balance
- range of motion
  &
- flexibility

- improving mobility/posture/muscle strength in lower body

According to research at, inter alia,
- *University of Miami* in Coral Gables, FL
- *University of Alabama*
  &
- *Birmingham VA Medical Center*
  (both in Birmingham, AL)
  as well as
- *University of Ottawa/Department of Rheumatology* in Ottawa,
  Canada

Also relieving depression and anxiety plus improving self-esteem,
according to research at *University of Leeds* in Leeds, UK.

Not to overlook that it may also relieve pain, according to *University of
California* in Los Angeles.

IN A NUTSHELL

The chronic/unsolved but debilitating health issue of Rheumatoid Arthritis
can well be relieved the natural way with different types of outdoor/aerobic
and indoor exercises. To manage swelling and inflammation of our joints,
also loss of muscle mass, etc. causing pain all over the body. Scientifically
validated. As indicated.

33. OSTEOPOROSIS: EXERCISE?

THE PHILOSOPHY BEHIND

In many cases, we may lose some 1% of bone density per year later in life (age 40+++). Potentially caused – inter alia - by
- unfavorable lifestyle (e.g., lack of physical exercise)
- unfavorable nutrition (e.g., sugary drinks)
- shortage of favorable nutrients (e.g., minerals magnesium/calcium/strontium/boron and/or vitamins A/B/C/D-3/E and/or estrogen, etc.)
- smoking
- emotional stress

Just to name some triggers...

Causing brittle bones leading to fractures in many cases.

Affecting some 3 million U.S. citizens.

Should you be (or a candidate for) one of those, fortunately, different kinds of exercise may well be the natural answer not only for relieve – but even for life extension. With special reference to...

PHYSICAL EXERCISING – SCIENTIFICALLY VERIFIED

...according to, inter alia, the *American Academy of Orthopedic Surgeons (AAOS)* in Rosemont, IL.

Let's start with

- ***Postural exercises***

to stretch and strengthen muscles in front (chest) and back of our body, cutting down the risk of spinal fractures.

With special reference to, inter alia, neck & head & full body stretches, as well as abdominal stretching

According to research at, inter alia,
- *University of Toronto* in Toronto, Canada
  and in South Korea at, inter alia,
- *Howon University* in Gunsan
- *Inje University* in Busan
- *Kimcheon Science College* in Gimcheon

To improve/maintain bone density, the U.S. *National Osteoporosis Foundation (NOF)* recommends 5-7 times the week

- ### *Weight bearing exercises*

For 30 minutes each. Potentially breaking up in 3 parts of 10 minutes each.

Unlike manifold assumptions, however, 'weight bearing' – according to *NOF* -does not only mean to carry any weights but also includes, inter alia,
- running
- playing tennis
- hiking
- jumping rope
- stair climbing
- dancing

Verified also by the U.S. *Bone Health and Osteoporosis Foundation* in Arlington, VA.

Not to shy away from

- ### *Muscle-strengthening exercises*

2-3 times a week, according to *NOF* by, inter alia,
- lifting additional weights (starting with light weights, increasing slowly)
- doing exercises for body weight (leg lifts/pushups)
- functional exercises (like rising on toes in standing position)
- applying elastic exercise bands

Especially, as these muscle-strengthening exercises for 30-60 minutes per week may have enormous

ADDITIONAL BENEFITS FOR OUR HEALTH & LIFE EXPECTANCY

By reducing the risk of those diseases topping the list of 'chronic' diseases with non-age-related premature mortality in our industrialized society according to the World Health Organization - heart disease, followed by cancer – and 10-20% of all-cause of mortality in general.

Based on research, inter alia, in Japan at
- *Tohoku University* in Sendai
- *Waseda University* in Tokyo
  &

-    *Kyushu University* in Fukuoka

Applying the muscle-strengthening exercise of 1 hour per week may also cut down the risk of diabetes. (#3 on the WHO of chronic diseases.) Based on same research.

Proving once again scientifically that our physical-mental-spiritual existence is a complex biologic-ecologic phenomenon with any part linked to others.

IN A NUTSHELL

Osteoporosis – lack of bone density causing brittle bones leading to fractures in many cases – are affecting 3 million U.S. citizens. Fortunately, certain physical exercises may not only decrease the risk considerably, but even the risk of top chronic diseases such as heart failure, cancer, and diabetes.

34. VITAMINS & MINERALS FOR YOUR HEALTH?

THE PHILOSOPHY BEHIND

As you know latest from our previous publications and seminars, your health depends primarily on healthy/balanced diet. Because of its inherent nutrients – with special reference to certain vitamins and minerals. As a basic requirement for specific vital tasks of our body and mind.

This requirement depends on our personalized metabolism. (Please note: 7 billion inhabitants of this planet the Earth have 7 billion individual metabolisms.) With special reference to factors like age, weight and overriding health condition generally.

Still, there are overriding guidelines we better understand and appreciate – to avoid debilitating disease and premature death.

Doing justice accordingly in favor of public health, the U.S. governmental *National Institutes of Health (NIH)* has worked out guidelines.

Supported by the independent nonprofit and non-governmental *National Institute of Sciences (NAS)* in Washington, D.C. Founded as an Act of Congress and approved by President Abraham Lincoln more than one and a half centuries ago in 1863.

VITAL VITAMINS & MINERALS

Following these guidelines, the U.S. governmental *Food and Drug Administration (FDA)* in Silver Spring, MD, has listed following vital vitamins and minerals. (Recommended daily intake as a minimum in brackets.)

Vitamins

- vitamin A (900 mcg)
- vitamin B-1 / thiamin (1.2 mg)
- vitamin B-2 / riboflavin (1.3 mg)
- vitamin B-3 / niacin (16 mg)
- vitamin B-5 / pantothenic acid (5 mg)
- vitamin B-6 (1.7 mg)

- vitamin B-7 / biotin (30 mcg)
- vitamin B-9 / folic acid (400 mcg)
- vitamin B-12 (2.4 mcg)
- vitamin C (90 mg)
- vitamin D (20 mcg)
- vitamin E (50 mg)
- vitamin K (120 mcg)
- choline (550 mcg)

Minerals

- calcium (1,300 mcg)
- magnesium (420 mg)
- iron (18 mg)
- potassium (4,700 mg)
- manganese (2.3 mg)
- copper (0.9 mg)
- phosphorus (1,250 mg)
- zinc (11 mg)
- selenium (55 mcg)
- chromium (35 mcg)
- iodine (150 mg)
- molybdenum (45 mcg)
- chloride (2,300 mg)
- sodium (2,300 mg)

DEFICIENCIES

While all of these vitamins and minerals are important for our health and well-being, there is quite some deficiency in our industrialized society. According to research at, inter alia, the *University of British Columbia* in Vancouver, Canada.

With special reference to
- vitamins A/B-6/B-12/C/D/E
  &
- minerals calcium/iron/magnesium

Just to pick the importance of the latter –

- ***magnesium**:*

This vital mineral is needed for no less but 600 (!) biochemical reactions in our body. According to research at *Radboud University Medical Center* in Nijmegen, The Netherlands.

In fact, there are many health issues caused by magnesium deficiency – of which more than 50% citizens of our 'modern' society are affected. I.e. with less than 0.75 millimoles per liter (mmol/l of magnesium in the blood.

Including
- blood sugar (diabetes)
- cognitive capability
- migraine headache
- kidney disease
  &
- health of muscles.
  In fact, magnesium is almost indispensable for well-functioning muscle contractions.

As verified scientifically at, inter alia,
- *Harvard School of Public Health* in Boston, MA
- *University of Hertfordshire* in Hartfield, UK
- *University of Palermo* in Palermo, Italy
- *University of Western Australia* in Perth, Australia

Finally not to forget about the impact of magnesium on our – yes - *longevity*.

According to research, inter alia, in California at the *University of California in Berkeley & Children's Hospital Oakland Research Institute* in Oakland.

IN A NUTSHELL

Besides physical activity, healthy diet is a basic prerequisite for good health and well-being. With specific nutrients in the forefront. Unfortunately yet, there are quite some deficiencies in terms of vitamins and minerals in our daily lifestyle we need to understand and counterbalance. To avoid being one of those 86% of non-age-related premature deaths in our country due to chronic/unsolved debilitating disease.

35. MEDITERRANEAN DIET FOR YOUR HEALTH?

THE PHILOSOPHY BEHIND

As you have learned from our previous blogs/publications/seminars, our life and well-being rests on 2 basic pillars: healthy diet and physical activity. As far as the first – healthy diet – is concerned, with special reference to a whole 'kingdom' of nutrients to support our body and mind.

While mankind has followed this blueprint of nature for millions of years, industrialization has tried to synthesize these laws of nature in many countries – with no overriding success.

Unlike those cultures staying within natural lifestyle – with special reference to their diet.

One of these cultures are in the Mediterranean region, i.e. north and south of the Mediterranean Sea where man lives already since millions of years in line with nature.

BASIC MEDITERRANEAN NUTRIENTS

Following traditional pattern, the Mediterranean diet consists basically of fresh plant foods such as a variety of
- fruits
- vegetables
  also
- legumes
  &
- whole grains
  also limited amounts of
- fish
  &
- dairy
  plus healthy fats such as
- seeds
- nuts
- olive oil
  but less
- white/red meat
  &

- eggs

Manifold surrounded by flavoring/tasty spices.

Today medically verified by, inter alia, the *American Heart Association.*

Vice-versa, the Mediterranean folks refrains widely from unhealthy 'Western diet' such as, inter alia,
- processed foods (like processed/deli meats & hot dogs, etc.)
- white flour/refined bread/pasta/pizza dough
- added sugar (like sodas/pastries/candies)
- trans fats (as in processed foods and margarines)

HEALTH BENEFITS – SCIENTIFICALLY VERIFIED

Fortunately, this Mediterranean diet is not only tasty – it has great benefits for our health and even longevity.

To pick 3 benefits as a small pattern, let's start with

- **_Cardiovascular disease_**

According to the *World Health Organization (WHO)* and the U.S. governmental *Centers for Disease Control and Prevention (CDC)* heart failure is leading global and U.S. statistics of premature (non-age-related) deaths.

Now we learn from research in Mediterranean Spain at, inter alia,
- *University of Barcelona & Hospital Clinic* in Barcelona
- *University of Valencia* in Valencia
- *University of Malaga* in Malaga
- *University of Navarra* in Pamplona
- *University of Las Palmas de Gran Canaria*
- *University of Balearic Islands* in Palma de Mallorca

that Mediterranean diet may well reduce the risk of heart attack, stroke – and related death – by 30%.

Same may be true for

- **_Weight loss_**

according to scientific research in the U.S. at, inter alia,

- *Harvard Medical School*
&

- *Brigham and Women's Hospital*
(both in Boston, MA)
and

- *Vanderbilt University School of Medicine* in Nashville, TN
with special reference to *hypertension*.

Also improvement of

- ### *Sleep quality*

May be well achieved according to research in Mediterranean country Greece at

- *Aristotle University of Thessaloniki* in Thessaloniki
- *University of Thessaly* in Larissa
&
- *Harokopio University* in Athens, the capital of Greece

Even more than that.

According to research in the U.S. at the

- *University of Illinois* in Urbana, IL
&
- *Harvard T.H. Chan School of Public Health* in Boston, MA
as well as international research at, inter alia,
- *University of Aberdeen* in Aberdeen
&
- *University of Oxford* in Oxford
(both UK)
and also the
- *University of Freiburg* in Freiburg, Germany
these very positive health effects (& more) of Mediterranean diet come specifically with *green* plant food.

IN A NUTSHELL

Mediterranean diet proves once more - scientifically verified - how important the kind of (natural) food is for our health and longevity. With special reference to green plant food we better may not overlook.

36. SUPPORT YOUR HEALTH WITH MANGOSTEEN?

THE PHILOSOPHY BEHIND

As you know latest from our publications and seminars, our life and health specifically depends – besides physical exercise – on what we are swallowing daily. With special reference to many different – yet powerful – plant-related nutrients. Without being vegetarian or even vegan.

Regardless, where we find those plants – domestic or exotic, i.e. in or outside our own country. What really counts is their nutritious power and diversity. Since man is created same way globally.

One of these exotic plants most of us may never have heard about is a small purple fruit named *mangosteen*. Native to countries like Thailand, the Philippines, Sri Lanka, Indonesia and Malaysia in Southeast Asia. Where it is used not only for nutrition but also as a traditional medicine.

With a taste familiar with that of strawberries/pineapples/peaches.

COMPREHENSIVE HEALTH BENEFIT – SCIENTIFICALLY VERIFIED

In terms of nutrients mangosteen is containing – as confirmed by the US. Department of Agriculture – inter alia
- vitamins A/B-6/B-9 (folate)/B-12/C/D
- minerals potassium/calcium/copper/manganese/zinc
- protein
- fiber

I.e., antioxidants which are manifold deficient in our Western diet.

Based on this diversity, we may not be surprised about its benefits also for us in the Western hemisphere where mangosteen is grown since a quarter of century also in Puerto Rico and Hawaii. Not only for pure nutrition but also for our health.

With special reference to the top of chronic diseases with manifold premature death, such as
- heart disease
- cancer
     &

- diabetes

Related to - sometimes chronic – inflammation which stands also behind
- depression
- arthritis
- Alzheimer's disease

According to research at, inter alia, the *University of Tsukuba* in Tsukuba, Japan.

IN A NUTSHELL

Mangosteen – a small purple fruit native to Southeast Asia (but grown meanwhile also in Puerto Rico & Hawaii) has many antioxidant and anti-inflammatory properties in favor of our health and longevity we may not want to overlook.

37. STRETCH FOR BETTER HEALTH!

THE PHILOSOPHY BEHIND

As we know from history – and natural medicine today – stretching can support and strengthen physical and mental power. In manifold ways. Proven by international research today.

HEALTH BENEFITS OF STRETCHING – SCIENTIFICALLY VERIFIED

- ***Back pain***

According to research in Finland at

- *University of Oulu*
  &
- *Oulu University Hospital*
  and
- *The Hong Kong Polytechnic University* in Hong Kong, China

stretching may well reduce lower back pain, and also improve range of motion.

Scientifically supported also by research in South Korea at, inter alia,

- *Inje University* in Gimhae
  &
- *Kyungnam University* in Changwon

- ***Headache***

Relieving headaches is another benefit of stretching (especially of upper back and neck), according to research in South Korea as well, at

- *Gachon University* in Incheon
  &
- *Sehan University* in Yeongamgun

with improving sound sleep as well.

- ***Mood & Cognitive Function***

Based on research at, inter alia, the

- *University of Electro-Communication* in Tokyo, Japan,

stretching can help to calm down and focus more precisely on tasks ahead.

Even for people who, otherwise, are not practicing physical exercise at all.

- ***Posture***

As we learn from research at, inter alia,

- *Universidade de Lisboa* in Portugal's capital Lisbon

regular stretching may well strengthen muscles, also encouraging alignment, thus improving our posture.

- ***Motion***

Both, dynamic and static stretching, may support muscle strength extend and reduce stiffness, thus improving bodily motion.

According to research at

- *Universite de Bourgogne-Franche-Comte* in Dijon, France

IN A NUTSHELL

Stretching – although practiced as one of traditional physical and mental activities since thousands of years – looks still 'maiden' for many in our modern time. This chapter may open briefly the window to at least a small sample of health benefits derived from stretching.

38. DIABETES – A MENTAL DISEASE?

THE PHILOSOPHY BEHIND

As you know, some 10% of the U.S. population is diabetic, with 1.5 million new diagnoses every year and a quarter of a million premature deaths.

Related to quite some physical problems. E.g., high blood glucose as the basic symptom of diabetes is also a risk factor for our heart with special reference to heart attack and stroke. As it may damage blood vessels and nerves which control our heart. Emphasizing the fact that heart disease and stroke are the leading causes of death.

However, this vicious cycle is not closed.

Appreciating the fact that man's existence is not one-dimensional but rather a complex biologic-ecologic phenomenon, diabetes' impact on our health is not only physically but rather mentally as well.

Let's focus on some

MENTAL IMPLICATIONS – SCIENTIFICALLY VERIFIED

according to U.S. governmental *Centers for Disease Control & Prevention (CDC)*, as verified also by the *British Diabetic Association* (also termed *Diabetes UK*).

With

- ***Diabetes distress***

on top as the overriding consequence of this disease. With typical symptoms such as, inter alia,
  - feeling of isolation
  - less motivation to manage the problem
  - making unhealthy choices

Affecting some
  - 20% of patients with diabetes type 2 & 25% with diabetes 1
    &

- one in 6 patients with non-insulin-dependent diabetes 2

Even worse, the existence of diabetes may have a tremendous negative effect on our

- ● ***Mood***

With respect to, inter alia,

- anxiety
- nervousness
- coordination
- irritability
- concentration
- aggression
- impatience
- confusion
- changes in personality/behavior
- making decisions
- feeling of tiredness/low energy or being unwell

According to professional evidence at, inter alia
- *Christus Santa Rosa Hospital* in San Antonio & New Braunfels, TX and research in Australia at
- *University of Melbourne* in Heidelberg/Parkville &
- *Flinders University* in Bedford Park

Another impact – according to the U.S. *National Institute of Diabetes and Digestive and Kidney Diseases* may be

- ● ***Depression***

due to lifestyle adjustments and changes of responsibilities when fighting diabetes.

With symptoms like, inter alia,
- disturbances/changes of sleep
- concentration problems
- nervousness
- energy loss
- missing interest in certain activities
- feeling of sadness or guilt

and sometimes even
- suicidal thoughts

Also in those cases where children/teenagers are affected and which can lead to, inter alia,
- worse performance at school
- irritability
- anger
- agitation
- abandonment of specific activities and/or friends

Also

- ***Anxiety***

may arise as the result of long-term management of diabetes.

According to research at, inter alia,
- *University of Toronto* in Toronto, Canada
  &
- *Universiti Kebangsaan Malaysia Medical Center (UKMMC)* in Kuala Lumpur, Malaysia

More than that, the mental impact of long-term management of diabetes, along with tensions and frustrations, can lead even to

- ***Disturbed relationship/marriage***

Including hampered sex life and erectile dysfunction.

Based on U.S. & international research at, inter alia,
- *Pennsylvania State University* at University Park, PA
- *Albert Einstein College of Medicine* in New York, NY
- *University of Delaware* in Newark, DE
- *University of Connecticut School of Medicine* in Farmington, CT
- *Nanyang Technological University* in Singapore

IN A NUTSHELL

Unlike manifold assumptions, diabetes as one of the most debilitating diseases in our society, does not come with a physical impact only. Rather, mental consequences of this health problem are of no less importance as indicated in this chapter.

39. HOW MANAGE IBS NATURALLY?

THE PHILOSOPHY BEHIND

Diet – healthy diet! – besides physical exercise – is the basic fundament of health and longevity by supporting our biologic-ecologic existence – body and mind. This, however, is not only a matter of satiety and taste. Rather, healthy diet requires many nutrients we better may not want to miss.

Disregarding this three-fold complexity may lead to debilitating digestive problems – affecting major part of our population. Medically termed 'Irritable Bowel Syndrome' (IBS).

With digestive symptoms such as
- constipation
- diarrhea
- bloating
- abdominal cramps

Additionally, symptoms may arise seemingly not being related to our digestion directly, like
- anxiety
- depression
- fatigue

Based on the physiological relationship between gut and brain.

I.e. that, independent of our diet, also mental issues like depression and stress may well play a role in creating IBS.

As indicated by the governmental U.S. *National Institute of Diabetes and digestive and Kidney Disease (NIDDK).*

NATURAL WAYS TO MANAGE IBS – SCIENTIFICALLY VERIFIED

This implies that, when thinking about management of IBS effects, we may focus certainly on our daily nutrition, but not only. Also on our daily lifestyle.

Dietary adjustments

Doing justice accordingly in terms of diet, to avoid and manage IBS best, basically 2 factors come to our mind, according to NIDDK: fiber and gluten.

- ***Fiber***

Thereby, 2 types of fiber are of relevance: soluble & insoluble fiber.

With priority of soluble fiber when it comes to managing constipation.

Available from nature inter alia, in
    - legumes (like beans/peas/lentils)
    - vegetables (like Brussels sprouts/carrots/broccoli/turnips)
    - fruits (like apples/grapefruit/oranges)
    - oat products

With special reference to *psyllium husk* – to be found in vegetables - which relieves constipation and abdominal pain, according to
    - *Baylor College of Medicine*
      &
    - *Texas Children's Hospital*
      (both in Houston, TX)

Doing justice, NIDDK recommends a daily input of 2-3 grams of psyllium husk with diet.

According to research at *Baylor College of Medicine, also swallowing of*

- ***Peppermint oil***

may relieve abdominal pain and IBS symptoms in general.

On the other hand,

- ***Gluten***

may be avoided or at least limited at the same time as this type of protein may worsen IBS symptoms according to NIDDK.

Therefore, it is recommended by NIDDK, to refrain as far as possible from gluten-rich diet such as
    - Processed foods (especially those which contain
      flavorings/colorings and thickening agents)

Lifestyle adjustments

E.g., with moderate

- ***Physical Exercise***

To
- improve constipation
- reduce abdominal bloating
  and also
- improve depression/anxiety/fatigue
  as well as to
- reduce stress

According to research at, inter alia,
- *University of Gothenburg* in Göteborg, Sweden
  as well as research in Iran at
- *Isfahan University of Medical Sciences* in Isfahan
  &
- *Ahvaz Jundishapur University of Medical Sciences* in Ahvaz

IN A NUTSHELL

No less but 10-20% of U.S. adults are affected by IBS (**I**rritable **B**owel **S**yndrome) as the most diagnosed digestive disorder of our seemingly modern times. Fortunately, nature gives us ways of self-therapy for relief. In terms of diet and lifestyle adjustments, as briefly focused on, scientifically validated.

40. ARE YOU IN GOOD EMOTIONAL HEALTH?

THE PHILOSOPHY BEHIND

As you know from our previous publications and seminars, our health is resting on 2 basic pillars: healthy diet and physical exercise. Only? Not at all. Appreciating the fact that we are biologically a complex phenomenon, there is one more factor related to our health: *emotions*.

WHAT IS EMOTIONS ALL ABOUT?

In fact, emotions are type of feeling which accompany our whole life in good or bad. With special reference to changes and challenges we are facing. Affecting both – our physical and our mental health. According to the *National Center for Emotional Wellness (NCEW)* in Melville, NY.

I.e., emotions are especially important when it comes to cope with stress in cases of difficult life-respective situations. Like
- changes in personal relationships
- problems at school or at work
- medical problems
- losing family/friends
which can well lead to health problems like raising blood pressure, undermining the immune system, and aggravating existing health issues.

According to research at, inter alia, *Laval University* in Quebec City, Canada.

Positive emotions, vice-versa, are important to support many life-respective situations especially for youngsters as well as seniors.

According to the U.S. *Centers for Disease Control and Prevention (CDC)* in cases of children/adolescents, e.g., to
- learn coping with problems
- learn appropriate social skills
- have good time at school and at home

Based on *National Health Service (NHS)* in the UIK, this effect can be supported in cases of youngsters by, inter alia,
- listen to them

- taking seriously what they say
- demonstrating interest in what they think

On the other hand, seniors with depression may well be candidates for, inter alia, lung disease, cardiovascular disease or arthritis.

According to research at, inter alia, *University College London* in London, UK.

In both cases – young and old – specific symptoms may point in direction of negative emotional development.

With youngsters, such as
- behavioral changes
  or
- difficulties to sleep

With seniors, such as
- difficulties to concentrate
- feeling of angriness
- fatigue
- mood swings
- feeling of restlessness
- missing interest in otherwise enjoying activities
- feelings of hopelessness/sadness
  or even
- thoughts of suicide/death

HOW IMPROVE EMOTIONAL HEALTH

Accordingly, it may be very helpful to support emotional wellness, just as the U.S. *National Institutes of Health (NIH)* with its 27 institutes and centers recommends with following strategies.

- **Stress reduction**

By, inter alia,
- regular exercise
- at least 7 hours of sleep at night
- times to relax
- focus on positive achievements

- **Improving social connections**

Inter alia by
- supporting relationships with friends and family
- learning from others about new things of joy
- joining clubs/groups with enjoyable activities

- ***Support positive mindset***

With, inter alia, healthy diet, exercise and sound sleep.

Just to indicate 3 examples.

IN A NUTSHELL

Right – healthy/balanced diet and physical exercise are the basic pillars our health is built on. Still, in order to strengthen this fundament of our life, *emotional* health plays a major role as well, as indicated above. Scientifically verified.

41. WHICH NUTRITION FOR LONGEVITY?

THE PHILOSOPHY BEHIND

As you know latest from our blogs/publications/seminars, healthy diet – besides physical exercise – is vital. Based on nutrients our nature is offering us, limitless. Depending on different qualities, quantities, and timings.

NUTRITIONAL BASICS FOR LONGEVITY – SCIENTIFICALLY VERIFIED

Although certain health factors such as age, genetics, sex, etc., play a basic role, certain nutrition is decisive for long and healthy life.

According to research at, inter alia,
- *Tufts University* in Boston, MA
- *University of Southern California* in Los Angeles, CA
- *Washington University School of Medicine* in St. Louis, MO &
- *Duke University School of Medicine* in Durham, NC

As a result of this extended research, following nutritional factors should dominate our diet: Inter alia,

- legumes
- whole grain
- calories up to 30% from olive oil and nuts
- white meat in a limited dimension
- no red/processed meat
- less sugar and refined carbohydrates
- 3 cycles of 5-day fasting/mimicking diet during the year
- day split (12 hours eating/12 hours fasting)

Additionally, keeping body mass index (BMI) under 25, may help very well.

Also, protein consumption should be adequate, especially beyond age 65 to avoid being malnourished, as seniors of this age could become frail with a low protein diet.

This is in line with research at

- *University of Bergen*
  &
- *Haukeland University Hospital*
  (both in Bergen, Norway)

According to which reduced consumption of red/processed meat (as a basic of Western diet) in favor of more legumes/whole grains/nuts may extend life for another 8 years beyond age 60.

With special reference to the fact that plant-based diet does not only cut down the risk of diabetes and cardiovascular disease but inflammation in general which, to be sure, is an underlying factor of any disease. With an impact on life extension, accordingly.

As scientifically verified also at the *Cleveland Clinic* in Cleveland, OH.

IN A NUTSHELL

Unlike Western diet, we should favor food rich in healthy nutrients such as legumes/whole grains/nuts/etc. and appropriate lifestyle including dietary time frame as well as weight control to extend life considerably. Scientifically verified by U.S. & international research.

42. UNFAVORABLE PLANTS FOR YOUR HEALTH?

THE PHILOSOPHY BEHIND

As you know latest from our publications and seminars, nature got the basics for our health and longevity. Including certain plants with appropriate nutrients and remedies. Still, there are plants in our cultivated backyards and gardens, as well as natural environments being counterproductive for our physical and mental wellbeing when, e.g., touched or eaten. Potentially leading not only to gastrointestinal upset but also to problems of our nervous system and even our heart - #1 of chronic disease in our industrialized society.

PLANTS COUNTERPRODUCTIVE FOR HEALTH – SCIENTIFICALLY VERIFIED

According to, inter alia, *University of Illinois College of Veterinary Medicine* in Urbana, IL, and *Northeast Ohio Medical University* in Rootstown, OH, verified by the U.S. *Centers for Disease Control and Prevention (CDC)* in Atlanta, GA (HQ) & Kampala, Uganda, poisonous plants, as to be found in many parts of North America, may be considered with caution in favor of our health.

Depending if these plants are touched – or eaten.

If touched, this may cause, inter alia,
- itching
- rash
- swelling
- streaking
- patches
- blisters

If eaten, the potential consequences may be, inter alia,
- high/low blood pressure
- dermatitis
- fast/slow heart rate
- nausea/vomiting
- fever
- headaches
- mental problems

- shortness of breath
- swellings
- blisters
- etc.

Just to take a small sample of 5 poisonous plants.

E.g.,

Oleander

Originally a native to the Mediterranean, is found today also in the U.S. at Lake Mead National Park in Nevada, the Death Valley National Park in California and in Hawaii. Planted in gardens and on roadside.

Although looking very nice with its colors red/orange/white/yellow, its substance *oleandrin* may well have an impact on heart function and even be lethal at higher dosage.

Jimson weed

is to be found in pastures and on roadside also of warm climates. With white or purple flowers.

Consuming it, can potentially have basically mental impact with respect to, inter alia,
- loss of consciousness
- dizziness/confusion
- hallucinations
- disorientation
- aggressive behavior

Giant hogweed

Its hollow stem contains a substance termed *noxious sap* not only causing potentially blistering of skin in situations of sunlight exposure but can also lead to (permanent/temporary) blindness when getting into the eyes.

Preferring cool areas with moisture, we find this plant, e.g., at
- on meadows
- rail tracks
- in ditches
- on roadsides

- along river banks
- etc.

Usually up to 15 ft tall and 3 ft wide. Visually appreciated because of their white flowers.

Poison hemlock

This plant, to be found usually in shady areas with moist soil at roadsides and/or marshes and pastures, can turn out comprehensively problematic for our health – if ingested.

As, in this case, it may not only cause muscle damage and tremors but harm kidneys and have a negative effect on the heart rate by slowing it down.

Manchineel

Basically found on the shores of tropical areas like in Florida with yellow-green flowers, when touched, it may cause itching, swelling, burning and blisters.

IN A NUTSHELL

Nature offers us a kingdom of plants – favorable & unfavorable for our health. This brief elaboration gives you at least an idea about some plants to watch out because of their potential negative impact on your health.

43. MANAGE OSTEOARTHRITIS NATURALLY

THE PHILOSOPHY BEHIND

According to U.S. *Centers for Disease Control and Prevention,* osteoarthritis (OA) is the leading version of arthritis in our civilization, affecting the joints of more than 32 million adult citizens – representing 10% of our total population. With special reference to pain and swelling of our knees, hips, and hands.

NATURAL ANSWERS – SCIENTIFICALLY VERIFIED

Although there is no cure, there are natural therapies, such as physical activities and changes of lifestyle to manage this debilitating health issue, as we shall briefly cover in following.

Let's start with

Heat/Cold Therapy

I.e. reducing pain and swelling of affected joints by applying heat and cold to those for reducing inflammation.

According to research at *Yasuj University of Medical Sciences* in Yasuj, Iran.

Applying the heat, e.g., by hot shower or 20 minutes hot tub and then warm compress.

And the cold by cold rub gel and/or cold compress around the respective joint.

Also

Physical Exercise

may help, with, inter alia, stretches such as
- quadriceps stretch
and
- hamstrings stretch
as well as

- swimming
- kick-backs
- recumbent cycling
- standing leg lifts
- sit and stand
- elliptical training

Mind-Body Approach

E.g. with exotic yoga & tai chi.

With special reference to hip and knee OA.

Based on research at, inter alia, the *University of Pennsylvania* in Philadelphia, PA & *Boston University School of Medicine* in Boston, MA.

Another exotic therapy is

Acupuncture

According to research at *Chengdu University of Traditional Chinese Medicine* in Chengdu, China.

To reduce pain and activate knee function.

An additional benefit in terms of lifestyle adjustments is

Healthy Diet

with special reference to

- *oily fish*

like sardines/mackerel/salmon

as well as

- *avocados & walnuts*

according to research at the *University of Surrey* in Guildford, UK.

IN A NUTSHELL

Osteoarthritis (OA) as the leading version of arthritis in our civilization, is affecting the hands/knees/hips of more than 10% of our population with swelling and pain of joints in knees/hips/hands. While there is no cure with synthetics causing side effects instead, nature may well relieve this vicious cycle.

44. OVERWORK – YOUR DEATH SENTENCE?

THE PHILOSOPHY BEHIND

Working for extended hours may well lead to professional and economic success. A situation we are familiar with from the past up to now. Still, there is some kind of new development we are facing since Corona pandemic has hit. Inter alia, geographically, as many preferred working at home to avoid infection by social distancing voluntarily, or as a kind of ordered lockdown. Working longer than 8 hours per day in many cases.

According to the U.S. *National Bureau of Economic Research* the length of average workdays extended almost 50 minutes as a result. Leading in many cases to *burnout*. With special reference to healthcare professionals and emergency responders. According to research at the *National University Health System* in Singapore.

Along with stress-related symptoms such as
- reduced efficacy professionally
- feeling of exhaustion
- feeling cynical or at least negative toward the job

according to the *World Health Organization (WHO)*.

And with unfavorable consequence on the health of our body and mind.

IMPACT ON HEALTH AND LIFE – SCIENTIFICALLY VERIFIED

Working longer per day and week may lead, inter alia, to

- **Depression**

as based on international research at, inter alia,
- *Karolinska Institutet* in Stockholm, Sweden
- *University of Parma* in Parma, Italy
  &
- *James Cook University* in North Queensland, Australia

Another potentially negative consequence may be

- **High blood pressure**

as based on research in the U.S. at the *Medical College of Wisconsin* in Milwaukee, Wisconsin.

Not to forget that this stress-related burnout may also be linked to

- ***Diabetes***

According to research in Netherland at
- *VU University Amsterdam* in Amsterdam
  &
- *Tilburg University* in Tilburg

As well as

- ***Digestive problems***

as identified at *l'Hôpital Saint-Eloi* in Montpellier, France
Also, this stress-related burnout may increase the production of the hormone cortisol in the body with the risk of

- ***Heart attack***

and

- ***Stroke***

according to scientific findings at
- *Lake Erie College of Osteopathic Medicine (LECOM)* in Bradenton, Florida
  &
- *Mary Fitzgerald Hospital* in Darby, Pennsylvania

More than that.

Based on research at, inter alia,
- *University of California* in Irvine, California
  &
- *Pennsylvania State University* in University Park, Pennsylvania
this situation may lead to premature

- ***Mortality***

As, according to *World Health Organization (WHO)*, working 55 hours per week or more may increase the risk of stroke by 35% and the risk of death from heart disease by 17%.

IN A NUTSHELL

Longer working days as triggered by COVID-19 pandemic may well have major impact on health and life, as indicated in this elaboration. Scientifically verified.

45. SAVE YOUR KIDS FROM ADHD NATURALLY

THE PHILOSOPHY BEHIND

According to U.S. *National Survey of Children's Health (NSCH)*, more than 6 million children in the country aged 2-17 are struck with ADHD, a neurodevelopmental health issue. Additional to more than 4% of adults suffering same problem. Verified by the U.S. *Centers for Disease Control and Prevention (CDC)*.

To put it in practical terms, these ADHD-related kids are fidget and hyperactive in permanent action such as running/climbing/jumping. Easily distracted from following instructions and paying attention.

Leading to inadequate social/academic/economic problems, increasing also the risk of injury and even hospitalization.

To get out of this seemingly vicious cycle, almost 2 thirds of these ADHD-struck kids are treated with synthetic drugs. Unfortunately, lacking appropriate success.

NATURE'S ANSWER – SCIENTIFICALLY VERIFIED

Only recently, *Ohio State University* in Columbus, OH, carried out a study with children aged 6-12 suffering ADHD, based on healthy diet with special reference to fruits and vegetables, to decrease ADHD symptoms.

Scientifically verified by, inter alia, at
- *University of Illinois* in Chicago, IL
  &
- *University of Central Arkansas* in Conway, AR

So far, so good – but which components of healthy food play a decisive role?

These are, inter alia, certain

Vitamins

like

- ***vitamin B-6***

As to be found in

- fish
- eggs
- potatoes
- peanuts

- ***vitamin D***

in

- fatty fish
- egg yolks
- beef liver
- fortified foods

Minerals

- ***magnesium***

Like in

- spinach
- pumpkin seeds
- peanuts
- almonds

- ***iron***

available in

- kidney beans
- liver
- beef
- tofu

- ***zinc***

as found in

- nuts
- beans
- shellfish

To cut down ADHD symptoms, also

Proteins

are recommended. In this case, we may consider as a source, inter alia,

- poultry products
- beans/lentils
- fish/shellfish
- nuts

Omega-3 fatty acids

Since ADHD-related children may be short in omega-3 fatty acids, research at the *Oregon Health and Science University* in Portland, Oregon, recommends to compensate with, inter alia, following foods in order to improve focus/attention/working memory/motivation:

- flax seeds
- chia seeds
- fatty fish (salmon/tuna)
- walnuts

IN A NUTSHELL

More than 6 million U.S. youngsters are struck with Attention Deficit Hyperactivity Disorder (ADHD). Nature offers relieve based on easily viable dietary adjustment.

46. SUFFER DIABETES? KNOW THE SYMPTOMS!

THE PHILOSOPHY BEHIND

According to the *World Health Organization (WHO)*, more than 80% of non-age-related mortality and more than ¾ of all ailments in our industrialized society are based on unsolved (chronic) diseases. With heart failure on top, followed by cancer and diabetes.

The latter, starting in most cases after age 45 and hitting a quarter of U.S. citizens aged 65 and over, comes with the disadvantage of not using the vital hormone insulin correctly in the body, to provide cells with appropriate energy to function. When blood sugar rises because of problems with use/production of insulin. Related to quite a few side effects leading to additional health issues – yes, a vicious cycle.

HOW REALIZE THIS PHENOMENON EARLY ENOUGH?

While it seems easy to verify this situation when going by the numbers, i.e. measuring blood sugar count technically, in order to counterbalance and avoid side effects in time, it is reasonable to realize the diabetic symptoms early enough. To fight this health issue in time.

According to, inter alia, U.S. federal agencies
- *National Heart, Lung and Blood Institute*
- *Centers for Disease Control and Prevention*
- *National Institute of Diabetes and Digestive and Kidney Diseases*

and U.S. medical research at, inter alia,
- *Weill Cornell Medical College* in New York
- *Mayo Clinic* in Rochester, Minnesota

These symptoms may be

- ***Fatigue***

In cases where cells are lacking glucose due to diabetic situation, the feeling of fatigue may arise.

- ***Infections/sores***

If blood circulation is poor, it takes more time to recover from infections and sores.

- ***Weight loss***

In cases of too little insulin, body may burn not only fat but also muscles for energy. Causing weight loss.

- ***More hunger***

Since organs and muscles are low on energy, as the cells cannot access glucose for energy in diabetic situation, one feels more hungry in this situation.

- ***Blurred vision***

Blood glucose too high may pull fluid from eye lenses leading to swelling with blurred vision temporarily.

- ***Frequent urination/increased thirst***

Also, if glucose is too high in the blood stream, body may extract fluid from tissues making more thirsty and more frequent urination.

Another early sign could be darkened skin on, e.g.
  - elbows
  - knuckles
  - armpits
  - groin
  - neck
  - knees
known by the medical term *acanthosis nigricans*.

IN A NUTSHELL

Since diabetes is one of the top chronic diseases in our industrialized society, it is important to realize in time its development. Know the symptoms - as indicated in this elaboration, verified by U.S. federal agencies and medical research, respectively.

47. HOW TACKLE UTI NATURALLY?

THE PHILOSOPHY BEHIND

Urinary tract infection (UTI) is not a death sentence. However, it is a very common issue of medical inconvenience in terms of bacterial infection. Prevalent in half of the female population at least once in life.

Based on research at, inter alia,
- *University College London* in London, UK
  &
- *University of Queensland* in Herston, Australia

With symptoms like, inter alia,
- urgency & increased frequency of urination
- cramping/pressure in lower abdomen/groin
- feeling of pain/burning during urination
- change of color/smell of urine
- bloody/cloudy/murky urine

Caused by the bacteria *escherichia coli*, with the consequence of cystitis as an inflammation.

To happen potentially as the result of
- diabetes
- sexual intercourse
- kidney transplant
  and
- antibiotics

The latter seeming 'schizophrenic', as antibiotics are the conventional medical way to treat this phenomenon. Yes, somehow a vicious cycle.

NATURAL WAYS TO OVERCOME UTI – SCIENTIFICALLY VERIFIED

Based on natural lifestyle adjustments as practiced by our ancestors for thousands of years, we can indeed take action successfully with quite a few and very simple home remedies and modalities, as follows.

Frequent urination

To flush the bacteria from the urination tract, don't hesitate to follow any urge for urination as soon as possible.

According to research at, inter alia, *Oakland University William Beaumont School of Medicine* in Auburn Hills, MI.

Hydration

To stay well hydrated is very important in this context, as the water you drink clears your body from waste, without flushing out vital nutrients.

At the same time the water is diluting the urine and the flush through the body is speeded up. Making it more difficult for the bacteria to infect the cells of urinary organs.

And how much water to drink for appropriate hydration?

6-8 glasses of 8 ounces per day. As suggested by the U.S. *National Institute of Diabetes and Digestive and Kidney Diseases* in Bethesda, MD & Phoenix, AZ.

Vitamin C

Additionally, ladies by the age of 19 plus may swallow at least 75 milligrams (men 90 mg) of Vitamin C daily, if they don't smoke. If they do, add 35 mg per day, both genders.

As recommended by the U.S. *National Institutes of Health* in Bethesda, MD, as this vitamin is reacting in urine with nitrates to create nitrogen oxides – killing bacteria.

Cranberry Juice

According to research at the *University of Sao Paulo* in Sao Paulo, Brazil, cranberry juice could prevent *escherichia coli* bacteria to cling to cells in the urinary tract and therefore recommends consuming some 400 milliliters of at least 25% cranberry juice per day.

Not to overlook

Sex Life

If it is not performed in good hygiene, it can lead bacteria into the urinary tract.

To avoid, do this before the intercourse, inter alia:
- washing genitals, primarily foreskin before and after intercourse
- use condom
- change condoms if changing from anal vaginal
- urinate shortly before/after sex
- both partners need to be aware of current/former UTI

According to U.S. *National Institute of Diabetes and Digestive and Kidney Diseases* in Bethesda, MD.

Finally

Probiotics

Unlike manifold assumptions, *bacteria* are not necessarily something bad. Rather, besides indeed 'bad' bacteria like those creating UTI (with no additional benefit at all), there are also 'good' bacteria – so called *probiotics* – killing the 'bad brother'.

In fact, there are probiotics of the *Lactobacillus* group to save our urinary tract from bad bacteria.

As scientifically verified inter alia at the *Government Medical College and Hospital* in Chandigarh, India.

By not only
- hindering bad bacteria to attach cells of the urinary tract but also
- developing the antibacterial *hydrogen peroxide* in urine &
- cut down the pH value of urine, thus creating a situation less favorable for bad bacteria

Where and how get the probiotics from?

In fact from healthy food, fermented or in dairy, such as
- sauerkraut
- yogurt
- certain types of cheese
- kefir

IN A NUTSHELL

Urinary Tract Infection (UTI), affecting some 50% of females sometimes in life, is seemingly a 'schizophrenic' medical issue. Based on – and saved by – bacteria. In this chapter you learned about the difference.

48. AYURVEDIC HERBS FOR YOUR HEALTH?

THE PHILOSOPHY BEHIND

As you know from our publications and seminars latest, our human existence is a biologic-ecologic phenomenon, strictly based on natural laws. So is our health and longevity. That's why conventional medicine can only suppress symptoms of disease – at best, along with side effects – but cannot cure.

As an example take mostly prescribed drug for diabetes worldwide which, according to its producer – a renowned international pharmaceutical company – has more than 5 dozens of side effects – but offers no cure.

Instead, the only thing which can support our health and longevity is our own natural immune system and self-healing power. With special reference to *medicinal herbs*. As we find them, e.g., in the Amazon rainforest, in colloquial language termed as the 'biggest natural pharmacy in the world', since man has entered this globe 2 ½ million years ago.

Based on this natural background, some 3000 years ago Ayurvedic medicine ('Ayurveda') has developed in India, based on nature's kingdom of plants. In order to balance our life, with special reference to detoxification of the body and physical as well as mental regeneration. With special reference to *medicinal herbs*.

Additional to other natural therapies such as dietary interventions and lifestyle adjustments.

While the list of diseases – especially chronic/unsolved health issues – is unlimited, let us pick as sample of debilitating chronic/unsolved diseases.

Like ...

Diabetes

to understand by this example the power of Ayurvedic herbs (additional to dietary interventions and lifestyle adjustments) which are known for *lowering glucose level* in diabetics. To be applied in different ways such as, inter alia, consuming the herbs as a tea.

With special reference to, inter alia, following herbs specifically and most (in alphabetical order):

- bitter melon
- fenugreek
- gymnema
- holy fruit tree
- Indian kino tree
- ivy guard
- margosa tree
- pomegranate
- tinospora
- turmeric

According to comprehensive Ayurvedic experience at
- *Ayurvaid Hospitals* in Bangaluru, India
  Verified by scientific research also in the U.S. in, inter alia,
  North Carolina at
- *Wake Forest University School of Medicine* in Winston-Salem
- *Duke University* in Durham
  &
- *University of North Carolina* at Chapel Hill
  As well as
- *Stanford University* in Stanford, CA
  &
- *Brown University* in Providence, RI

Gastritis

is another health issue with Ayurvedic herbs helping to lead the way out of
debilitation. By offering anti-inflammatory/antioxidant/antiulcer effect.

Based on Ayurvedic herbs such as, inter alia,
- licorice
- ginger
- panax ginseng
- peepal tree
- bael tree
- heartleaf hemp vine

According to research at, inter alia, *Tabriz University of Medical Sciences*
in Tabriz, Iran.

Constipation

For this rather common health issue of our time with, inter alia, lots of processed foods and lack of physical activity,

- ***Triphala***

has come to scientific limelight as an Ayurvedic laxative appropriate for gastrointestinal issues.

Based on research at, inter ala,
- *University of California San Diego School of Medicine* in La Jolla
- *Bastyr University* in San Diego
  &
- *Chopra Foundation, Department of Ayurveda and Yoga Research* in Carlsbad
  (all 3 in California)

In fact, it is a blend of plants such as *Amalaki* (emblica officinalis), *Haritaki* (terminalia chebula), and *Bibhitaki* (terminalia bellerica).

Similar effective is the Ayurvedic herb

- ***Senna***

to relieve constipation, when taken no longer than one week, as it stimulates the lining of the bowel, thus causing bowel movement within 6-12 hours.

According to the *American Society of Health System Pharmacists* in Bethesda, MD.

Gastroesophageal Reflux Disease (GERD)

According to research in Italy at, inter alia,
- *University of Catania* in Catania
- *Universita Di Messina* in Messina
  &
- *Societa Italiana di Medicina Generale* in Firenze
certain Ayurvedic herbs can treat causes, as well as manage the symptoms of gastroesophageal reflux disease (GERD) such as, inter alia,
- rosemary
- ginger
- aloe vera leaf gel
- marshmallow
- slippery elm

- Asian wormwood
- celandine
- belladonna/deadly nightshade
- carob
- turmeric
- fumitory-of-the-wall

Not to overlook the power of Ayurvedic herbs in terms of

Erectile dysfunction
(ED)

The essential oil of

- ***Cinnamomum cassia***

being one of those.

By relaxing erectile tissues. To be applied to the skin or inhaled via aromatherapy, after dilution in a carrier oil.

According to research in Turkey's capital Ankara at, inter alia,
- *Ankara University*
- *Cukurova University*
  &
- *Ankara Numune Education and Research Hospital*
as well as in Croatia at the
- *University of Split* in Split

With

- ***Ashwagandha***

being another powerful Ayurvedic herb in this case, native to India, the Middle East and partly in Africa.

According to, inter alia, *Ayurvedic Medical College & Hospital* in Agra, India.

IN A NUTSHELL

When it comes to support of health and longevity, besides of healthy diet and physical activity medicinal herbs play a decisive role on top. Since thousands of years – like Ayurvedic herbs. Scientifically verified today.

49. DIABETICS: KNOW VICIOUS COMORBIDITIES

THE PHILOSOPHY BEHIND

As you know from our previous studies, according to World Health Organization (WHO) statistics, 86% of non-age-related deaths and 77% of diseases in general are the consequence of chronic (unsolved) diseases. With heart failure, cancer and diabetes 2 on top.

Not only this. Diabetes is also related to quite a few debilitating comorbidities you should know in case you are affected. So are ¾ of diabetics with at least one comorbidity, and 44% with at least 2 comorbidities.

According to comprehensive research in the UK at, inter alia,
- *University of Manchester* in Manchester
- *University of Oxford* in Oxford
- *University of Nottingham* in Nottingham
- *University of Sussex* in Brighton
  &
- *Keele University* in Staffordshire

With similar scientific results in Asia at, inter alia,
- *Hokkaido University* in Sapporo, Japan
  &
- *National University of Singapore* in Singapore

To start with

Heart Disease

This is not only on top as #1 of the above mentioned chronic/unsolved diseases on the WHO list, but also related to diabetes.

As diabetes affects in a negative way the nerves and blood vessels supporting our heart, hardening the arteries.

That's why 30% of diabetics are affected by heart disease and/or stroke – with the risk of heart failure - according to the U.S. governmental *Centers for Disease Control and Prevention (CDC)*.

In this case the heart may not work efficiently to pump blood, as it is supposed to do.

Related to other health issuers like buildup of fluid in lungs, with difficulty of breathing, and swelling in legs.

That's why cardiovascular events, including stroke and heart attack leading to main cause of premature death, are not uncommon for diabetics.

In this context we have also to see that

Hypertension

is one of these comorbidities.

This can happen as the raised blood sugar in cases of diabetes damages blood vessels increasing the resistance in arteries leading to higher blood pressure.

As based on research at, inter alia, *Kagoshima University* in Kagoshima, Japan.

In fact, according to
- *Tulane University* in New Orleans, LA
   &
- *Peking University Health Science Center* in Beijing, China

more than 85% of diabetics are affected by hypertension.

Kidney Disease

is another potential consequence if diabetes 2, especially as the role of kidneys is related also to blood pressure regulation.

High blood sugar may also have a negative effect on the blood vessels of the kidneys. According to the U.S. *National Institute of Diabetes and Digestive and Kidney Diseases (NIDDK)*.

Leading to the fact that diabetes is the primary cause of kidney failure, according to the U.S. *National Kidney Foundation*.

Sleep Disorders

Around half of diabetics, if not even up to 3 quarters, are struck by sleep problems. Based on blood sugar irregularities.

According to research in the U.S. at the
- *University of Illinois* in Chicago, IL
  &
- *University of Delaware* in Newark, DE
  as well as in China at
- *Shanghai Jiaotong University* in Shanghai

Waking up several times at night for urination and otherwise.

Along with sleep disorders such as, inter alia,

- Insomnia
  i.e problems of
  - falling asleep
  - staying asleep
  - finding sound sleep

- Restless leg syndrome
  I.e. sensations in the leg

- Sleep apnea
  I.e. breathing irregularities on and off during the sleep

Also, it is possible that diabetics develop certain types of

Cancer

like, inter alia
- breast
- colon
- pancreatic
- liver
- bladder
cancer.

Based on complexity of related diabetic health issuers such as, inter alia,
- inflammation
- insulin resistance
  &
- overestimated cell growth

According to research in Saudi Arabia at
- *Princess Nourah bint Abdulrahman University* in Riyadh
  &

-    *Prince Sultan Military Medical Center* in Sulimaniyah

Obesity

I.e. being heavily overweight like 90% of diabetics are, is also crucial in context with diabetes.

As this correlation may be involving high level of lipids to impair function of pancreas, thus producing less insulin, leading to insulin resistance because of the higher level of lipids.

Based on experience at *Royal London Hospitals* in London, UK.

Not to forget that conventional treatment of diabetes including, inter alia, dosing of insulin, monitoring of blood sugar and blood sugar and meal planning can lead to

Mental Problems

such as, inter alia,
-    anxiety
-    depression
-    stress
-    anger
     and erven
-    suicidal ideation

according to the U.S. *Centers for Disease Control and Prevention (CDC)*.

IN A NUTSHELL

Diabetes 2 is not only one of the chronic/unsolved health problems of our time, it is also related to at least one crucial comorbidity in 3 quarters of cases. Scientifically validated.

50. PREVENT OSTEOARTHRITIS / OSTEOPOROSIS?

THE PHILOSOPHY BEHIND

At first glance, there is no difference between osteoarthritis & osteoporosis. Since both health issues are affecting our musculoskeletal system. I.e. – to be more precise – our bones/cartilage/joints/muscles/ligaments.

Not only this, both medical issues have same impact in terms of pain, as well as on social and the quality of life in general.

While, statistically, both conditions happen in second half of life, osteoporosis is more frequent in females. Although younger people may also be affected by osteoarthritis in case they have a genetic defect of their cartilage.

LEARN ABOUT THE DIFFERENCE – BASED ON SCIENTIFIC EVIDENCE

Still, there is a difference between both osteopathic conditions you should know in case you are affected by one of those.

According to research at, inter alia, the *International Islamic University Malaysia (IIUM)* in Kuala Lumpur, Malaysia and *Gazi University* in Turkey's capital of Ankara.

With special reference in the U.S. according to the governmental *National Institute of Arthritic and Musculoskeletal and Skin Disease.*

OSTEOARTHRITIS

Unlike osteoporosis which affects the strength and consistency of our bones, osteoarthritis may also change the shape of our bones. Yet, basically it is related to potential breakdown of our *joints*.

Symptoms

Coming up with symptoms such as, inter alia,
- reduced motion
- stiffness (mostly already in the morning)
- aches/pain of joints
- swelling of joints

- buckling/instability of joints
- popping/clicking sound in joints

Related to

Risks

(besides of genetics) such as, inter alia,
- poor alignment of joints/bone structure
- weak muscles (may also cause poor alignment)
- overuse/injury or joints
- obesity
- female gender
- lack of physical activity
- unhealthy diet
- age beyond 50

OSTEOPOROSIS

This medical situation becomes relevant when the bones are getting brittle to break, quicker than the body can rebuild it.

Symptoms

To be realized partly right at the beginning, there are potential symptoms.

Such as, inter alia,
- broken bone
- hump in upper back
- back pain, potentially indicating a vertebral or compression
- fracture
- loss of height
- tooth loss (if the jaw is affected)

Risks

And what are the risks of being struck by osteoporosis?

Potentially, inter alia

- medications like antiseizure drugs or corticosteroids
- lack of physical exercise
- genetically small body frames

- family history of osteoporosis
- medical conditions like celiac disease or after hysterectomy (to remove ovaries)
- females after menopause or during menopause before age 45
- males with low levels of testosterone
- smoking or high alcohol consumption
- being of Asian ancestry

PREVENT OSTEOARTHRITIS/OSTEOPOROSIS NATURALLY

To avoid **osteoarthritis**

- *physical exercise*

is recommended with 30 minutes daily/5 times a week to
- strengthen muscles supporting the joints
  &
- keep them flexible

Also, manage

- *weight control*

to avoid cartilage breakdown in knees and hips due to overweight/obesity.

Not to overlook to

- *regulate blood sugar*

as high blood sugar (diabetes!) can stiffen cartilage and even lose it.

Finally, apply

- *lifestyle adjustments*

  such as
- non-smoking
- stress management
- sound sleep
- avoiding alcohol abuse

To prevent **osteoporosis**

there are similar lifestyle adjustments recommended, as follows.

- non-smoking
- weight-bearing exercise (jogging/dancing/hiking)
- other physical exercise
- avoiding alcohol abuse
- eat a balanced diet (including vitamin D & calcium)

IN A NUTSHELL

Both – osteoarthritis & osteoporosis – are our most 'modern' musculoskeletal diseases affecting our bones and joints. They are still different to understand – and to prevent. Scientifically verified. Read on to learn about the details.

INDEX: HEALTH CONDITIONS & NATURAL REMEDIES / MODALITIES

(Alphabetical Order / Chapter Number)

REFERENCES: U.S. & INTERNATIONAL MEDICAL SCHOOLS / INSTITUTIONS

(Alphabetical Order / Chapter Number)

<u>U.S.A.</u>

Albert Einstein College of Medicine (New York, NY) 38
American Academy of Orthopedic Surgeons (Rosemont, IL) 33
American Society of Health System Pharmacists (Bethesda, MD) 48
Andrews University (Berrien Springs, MI) 30
Augusta University/Medical College of Georgia (Augusta, GA) 2
Avalon University School of Medicine (Girard, OH) 13
Bastyr University (San Diego, CA) 48
Baylor College of Medicine (Houston, TX) 39
Binghamton University (Binghamton, NY) 24
Boston University (Boston, MA) 14
Boston University School of Medicine (Boston, MA) 43
Brigham and Women's Hospital (Boston, MA) 2/7/35
Brown University (Providence, RI) 48
California Dairy Research Foundation (Davis, CA) 30
California Institute of Behavioral Neurosciences and Psychology (Fairfield, CA) 13
California State University (Hayward, CA) 17
Children's Hospital Oakland Research Institute (Oakland, CA) 23/34
Chopra Foundation, Department of Ayurveda and Yoga Research (Carlsbad, CA) 48
Christus Santa Rosa Hospitals (San Antonio & New Braunfels, TX) 38
City University of New York (New *ley* York City, NY) 1
Cleveland Clinic (Cleveland/Lyndhurst, Ohio) 2/41
Columbia University (New York, NY) 15
Duke University School of Medicine (Durham, NC) 41/48
Florida State University (Tallahassee, FL) 5
Harvard Medical School (Boston, MA) 2/7/8/16/35
Harvard School of Public Health (Boston, MA) 2/3/7/8/10/23/30/34
Harvard T.H. Chan School of Public Harvard Health (Boston, MA) 2/35
Homestead Hospital (Homestead, FL) 20
Hypertension Institute (in Nashville, TN) 10
Institute for Functional Medicine (Federal Way, WA) 21
Johns Hopkins Hospital (Tampa, FL) 20
Johns Hopkins University (Baltimore, MD) 28
Lake Erie College of Osteopathic Medicine (Bradenton, FL) 44
Lehman College (West Bronx, NY) 8
Louisiana State University System (Baton Rouge, LA) 2/14
Loyola University Chicago (Maywood, IL) 8/31
Mary Fitzgerald Hospital (Darby, PA) 44
Mayo Clinic (Rochester, MN) 31/46
Medical College of Wisconsin (Milwaukee, WI) 44
Mount Sinai Medical Center (Miami Beach, FL) 29

University of Tennessee (Knoxville, TN) 11
University of Texas Southwestern Medical Center (Dallas, TX) 8
University of Washington (Seattle, WA) 1/24/28
University of Western States (Portland, OR) 21
Vanderbilt University School of Medicine (Nashville, TN) 35
Veterans Affairs Medical Center (Tuscaloosa, AL) 6/14
Wake Forest University School of Medicine (Winston-Salem, NC) 48
Washington University School of Medicine (St. Louis, MO) 2/41
Wayne State University School of Medicine (Detroit, MI) 31
Weill Cornell Medical College/Center (New York, NY) 20/46

INTERNATIONAL

Aarhus University (Aarhus, Denmark) 5
Abant Izzel Bay Sal University (Bolu, Turkey) 8
Agha Khan University (Karachi, Pakistan) 25
Ahvaz Jundishapur University of Medical Sciences (Ahvaz, Iran) 39
Alexandria University (Alexandria, Egypt) 22
American University of Beirut (Beirut, Lebanon) 22
Andhra University (Andhra Pradesh, India) 1
Ankara Numune Education and Research Hospital (Ankara, Turkey) 48
Ankara University (Ankara, Turkey) 48
Arctic University (Tromso, Norway) 11
Aristotle University of Thessaloniki (Thessaloniki, Greece) 35
Aslang Ayurveda Hospital and Research Centre (Kathmandu, Nepal) 27
AyurVAID Hospitals (Bangaluru, India) 48
Ayurvedic Medical College & Hospital (Agra, India) 48
Bandirama Omyedi Eylul University (Bandirama, Turkey) 5
Breast Cancer Now (London, UK) 25
Canakkale Onsekiz Mart University (Canakkale, Turkey) 21
Capital Medical University (Beijing, China) 15
Central Queensland University (Melbourne, Australia) 15
Chalmers University of Technology (Goeteborg, Sweden) 5
Chengdu University of Traditional Chinese Medicine (Chengdu, China) 43
Chinese Academy of Medical Sciences (Beijing, China) 19
Chonbuk National University (Jeonju, South Korea) 14
City University London (London, UK) 17
CSIR-Indian Institute of Chemical Technology (Hyderabad, India) 16
Cukurova University (Ankara, Turkey) 48
Cyprus University of Technology (Lemesos, Cyprus) 21
Dalian University of Technology (Dalian, China) 1
Danube University of Krems (Krems, Austria) 29
Dongying People's Hospital (Dongying, China) 19
Far Eastern Federal University (Vladivostok, Russia) 18
Fatih University (Istanbul, Turkey) 7
Federal University of Rio Grande do Sul (Porto Alegre, Brazil) 8/24
Flinders University (Bedford Park, Australia) 38
Gachon University (Incheon, South Korea) 37
Gazi University (Ankara, Turkey) 5/50
Government Medical College (Kozhikode/Banda, India) 4

Government Medical College and Hospital (Chandigarh, India) 47
Griffith University (Gold Coast, Australia) 15
Grigore T. Popa University of Medicine and Pharmacy (Lasi, Romania) 6
Guilin Medical University (Guilin, China) 19
Gukurova University (Adana, Turkey) 5
Hallym University College of Medicine (Anyang, South Korea) 15
Hankuk University of Foreign Studies (Seoul, South Korea) 6
Hannam University (Daejeon, South Korea) 16
Harbin Medical University (Harbin, China) 1
Harokopio University (Athens, Greece) 35
Haukeland University Hospital (Bergen, Norway) 41
Heart and Diabetes Center North Rhine-Westphalia (Oeynhausen, Germany) 26
Heinrich-Heine-University (Düsseldorf, Germany) 14
Hokkaido University (Sapporo, Japan) 49
Hong Kong Polytechnic University (Hong Kong, China) 29/37
Hôpital Saint-Eloi (Montpellier, France) 44
Hospital del Mar Medical Research Institute (Barcelona, Spain) 13
Hospital Universitari de Sant Joan de Reus (Reus, Spain) 2
Howon University (Gunsan, South Korea) 33
Huazhong University of Science and Technology (Wuhan, China) 2/10
Hunan University of Chinese Medicine (Changsha, China) 19
Imperial College London (London, UK) 5
Inje University/College of Medicine (Busan/Gimhae/Gyeongsangnam-do/Seoul, South Korea) 5/33/37
Institute of Food Science and Technology and Nutrition (Madrid, Spain) 30
International Islamic University Malaysia/IIUM (Kuala Lumpur, Malaysia) 50
Isfahan University of Medical Sciences (Isfahan, Iran) 39
Istanbul Yeni Yuzyil University (Istanbul, Turkey) 22
James Cook University (North Queensland, Australia) 44
Jan Kochanowski University (Kielce, Poland) 10
Jeonju University (Jeonju, South Korea) 8
Josip Juraj Strossmayer University of Osijek (Osijek, Croatia) 24
Kagoshima University (Kagoshima, Japan) 49
Karelia University of Applied Sciences (Joensuu, Finland) 11
Karolinska Institutet (Stockholm, Sweden) 44
Kasturba Medical College (Manipal, India) 13
Keele University (Keele/Staffordshire, UK) 18/49
Keio University School of Medicine (Tokyo, Japan) 29
Kimcheon Science College (Gimcheon, South Korea) 33
King Abdulaziz University (Jeddah, Saudi Arabia) 29
King Georgia's Medical University (Lucknow, India) 19
King's College (London, UK) 30
Kobe University (Kobe, Japan) 1
Kyoto Prefectural University of Medicine (Kyoto, Japan) 10
Kuopio University Hospital (Kuopio, Finland) 29
Kyungnam University (Changwon, South Korea) 37
Kyushu University (Fukuoka, Japan) 33
Laval University (Quebec City, Canada) 40
Lebanese International University (Beirut, Lebanon) 22
London Sleep Centre-Neuropsychiatry (London, UK) 15
Luliu Hatiegano University of Medicine and Pharmacy (Cluj-Napoca, Romania) 21

Lund University (Lund, Sweden) 30
Mahidol University (Bangkok, Thailand) 9
Maulana Azad Medical College (New Delhi, India) 4/31
McMaster University (Hamilton, Canada) 2
Memorial University of Newfoundland (St. John's, Canada) 31
Monash University (Melbourne, Australia) 19
Mugla Sitki Kocman University (Mugla, Turkey) 25
MVR Cancer Center & Research Institute (Kerala, India) 25
Nanchang University (Nanchang, China) 22
Nanjing Jinling Hospital (Nanjing, China) 19
Nanyang Technological University (Singapore) 38
National University Health System (Singapore) 44
National University of Singapore (Singapore) 8/49
Newcastle University (Newcastle upon Tyne, UK) 13
Ottawa Hospital (Ottawa, Canada) 28
Oulu University Hospital (Oulu, Finland) 37
Pai Chai University (Daejeon, South Korea) 6
Peking Union Medical College (Beijing, China) 19
Peking University Health Sciences Center (Beijing, China) 30/49
People's Hospital of Ningxiang (Ningxiang, China) 9
Pomeranian Medical University (Szczecin, Poland) 17
Population Health Research Institute/PHRI (Hamilton, Canada) 2
Prince Sultan Military Medical Center (Sulimaniyah, Saudi Arabia) 49
Princess Nourah bint Abdulrahman University (Riyadh, Saudi Arabia) 49
Pusan National University (Busan, South Korea) 29
Queen Mary's University (London, UK) 30
Radboud University Medical Center (Nijmegen, The Netherlands) 34
Royal Hobart Hospital (Hobart, Australia) 19
Sapienza University of Rome (Rome, Italy) 23
School of Allied Health Sciences (Manipal, India) 13
Second Affiliated Hospital of Nanchang University (Nanchang, China) 22
Sehan University (Yeongamgun, South Korea) 37
Seonam University (Namwon, South Korea) 14
Seoul National University College of Medicine (Seoul, South Korea) 15
Service Institute of Medical Sciences (Lahore, Pakistan) 25
Sf. Spiridon Emergency Hospital (Iasi, Romania) 14
Shahid Beheshti University of Medical Sciences (Tehran, Iran) 24
Shandong University (Jinan, China) 10/14
Shanghai Jiaotong University (Shanghai, China) 49
Sheffield Hallam University (Sheffield, UK) 30
Shenzhen University School of Medicine (Schenzhen, China) 2
Sichuan University (Chengdu, China) 24
South China Agricultural University (Guangzhou, China) 1
Southeast University (Nanjing, China) 8
Spanish Medical Research Centre in Diabetes and Associated Metabolic Disorders (Madrid, Spain) 30
State University of Maringa (Maringa, Brazil) 19
Stockholm University (Stockholm, Sweden) 19
Stockport NHS Foundation Trust (Stockport, UK) 25
Tabriz University (Tabriz, Iran) 16/48

Technical University (Munich, Germany) 8
Technical University of Denmark (Kongens Lyngby, Denmark) 5
Tezpur University (Napaam, India) 22
Tilburg University (Tilburg, The Netherlands) 44
Tohoku University (Sendai, Japan) 33
Tongji University School of Medicine (Shanghai, China) 10
Turgut Özal University (Ankara, Turkey) 7
Ulster University (Londonderry, UK) 11
Umea University (Umea, Sweden) 11
Universidad de Santiago de Chile (Santiago, Chile) 52
Universidad Nacional de Colombia (Bogota, Colombia) 8
Universidade da Beira Interior (Covilha, Portugal) 14
Universidade de Lisboa (Lisbon, Portugal) 37
Universidade Federal de Goias (Goias, Brazil) 16
Universidade Federal do Maranhao (Maranhao, Brazil) 15
Universita Di Messina (Messina, Italy) 48
Universita Vita-Salute San Raffaele (Milan, Italy) 2
Universitario Son Espases (Palma de Mallorca, Spain) 7
Universitat Rovira I Virgili (Reus, Spain) 7
Universite de Bourgogne-Franche-Comte (Dijon, France) 37
Universite Laval (Quebec City, Canada) 5
Universiti Kebangsaan Malaysia Medical Center (Kuala Lumpur, Malaysia) 29/38
Universiti Putra Malaysia (Selangor Darul Ehsan, Malaysia) 29
University College Cork (Cork, Ireland) 11
University College London (London, UK) 40/47
University Hospital Center 'Mother Theresa' (Tirana, Albania) 20
University Hospital Lausanne (Lausanne, Switzerland) 22
University Medical Center Utrecht (Utrecht, The Netherlands) 5
University of Aberdeen (Aberdeen, UK) 2/29/30/35
University of Agricultural Sciences and Veterinary Medicine (Cluj-Napoca, Romania) 21
University of Antioquia (Medellin, Colombia) 8
University of Auckland (Auckland, New Zealand) 5/9
University of Balearic Islands (Palma de Mallorca, Spain) 35
University of Barcelona (Barcelona, Spain) 2/7
University of Bari (Bari, Italy) 20
University of Belgrade (Belgrade, Serbia) 9
University of Bergen (Bergen, Norway) 41
University of Bologna (Bologna, Italy) 29
University of Bonn (Bonn, Germany) 24/26
University of British Columbia (Vancouver, Canada) 34
University of Cambridge (Cambridge, UK) 2/8/31
University of Catania (Catania, Italy) 48
University of Chinese Academy of Sciences Shenzhen Hospital (Shenzhen, China) 2
University of Colombo (Colombo, Sri Lanka) 1
University of Copenhagen (Frederiksberg, Denmark) 5/8
University of East Anglia (Norwich, UK) 2/14
University of Eastern Finland (Kuopio, Finland) 29
University of Edinburgh (Edinburgh, UK) 18
University of Electro-Communication (Tokyo, Japan) 37
University of Florence (Florence, Italy) 31

University of Freiburg (Freiburg, Germany) 35
University of Gothenburg (Gothenburg/Göteborg, Sweden) 19/39
University of Granada (Granada, Spain) 13
University of Guelph (Guelph, Canada) 21
University of Hertfordshire (Hartfield, UK) 23/34
University of Insubria (Varese, Italy) 20
University of Kragujevac (Kragujevac, Serbia) 6
University of Kuopio (Kuopio, Finland) 8
University of Las Palmas de Gran Canaria (Las Palmas, Spain) 2/7/35
University of Latvia (Riga, Latvia) 31
University of Laval (Quebec City, Canada) 13
University of Leeds (Leeds, UK) 30
University of Liverpool (Liverpool, UK) 30
University of 'Magna Graecia' of Catanzaro (Catanzaro, Italy) 20
University of Malaga (Malaga, Spain) 2/7/35
University of Manchester (Manchester, UK) 4/28/49
University of Mauritius (Reduit, Mauritius) 18
University Medical Center Utrecht (Utrecht, The Netherlands) 14
University of Medicine (Tirana, Albania) 20
University of Medicine and Pharmacy (Iasi, Romania) 14
University of Melbourne (Heidelberg/Parkville/Melbourne, Australia) 38
University of Milan (Milan, Italy) 20
University of Montenegro (Podgorica, Montenegro) 9
University of Montreal (Montreal, Canada) 14
University of Naples Federico II (Portici, Italy) 5/21
University of Navarra (Pamplona, Spain) 2/7/35
University of Newcastle (New Lambton, Australia) 24
University of New South Wales (Kensington, Australia) 24
University of Nottingham (Nottingham, UK) 8/49
University of Oslo (Oslo, Norway) 19/29
University of Otago (Christchurch, New Zealand) 10
University of Ottawa (Ottawa, Canada) 27
University of Oulu (Oulu, Finland) 38
University of Oxford (Oxford, UK) 4/17/30/35/49
University of Palermo (Palermo, Italy) 1/23/34
University of Parma (Parma, Italy) 44
University of Pretoria (Pretoria, South Africa) 25
University of Queensland (St. Lucia, Australia) 19/27/28/47
University of Rome (Rome, Italy) 31
University of Sao Paulo (Sao Paulo, Brazil) 47
University of Singapore (Singapore) 18
University of South Australia (Adelaide, Australia) 5/26
University of South China (Hengyang, China) 19
University of Split (Split, Croatia) 48
University of Surrey (Guildford, UK) 43
University of Sussex (Brighton, UK) 49
University of Sydney (Sydney, Australia) 4
University of Tasmania (Tasmania, Australia) 19
University of Thessaly (Larissa/Magnisia, Greece) 21/35
University of Tokyo (Tokyo, Japan) 17

University of Tromso (Tromso, Norway) 5
University of Torino (Torino, Italy) 27
University of Toronto (Toronto, Canada) 16/33/38
University of Tsukuba (Tsukuba, Japan) 36
University of Valencia (Valencia, Spain) 2/7/35
University of Western Australia (Perth/Crawley, Australia) 23/31/34
University of Zagreb (Zagreb, Croatia) 16
University of Zurich (Zurich, Switzerland) 15
University Paris-Saclay (Villejuif, France) 5
Vendome Hospital (Vendome, France) 28
Vrije Universiteit Amsterdam (Amsterdam, The Netherlands) 14
Vrije Universiteit Brussel (Brussels, Belgium) 20
VU University Medical Center (Amsterdam, The Netherlands) 14/44
Wageningen University (Wageningen, The Netherlands) 6
Waseda University (Tokyo, Japan) 33
Yasuj University of Medical Sciences (Yasuj, Iran) 43
Yonsei University (Wonju, South Korea) 6
Zanjan University of Medical Sciences (Zanjan, Iran) 17
Zhejiang University (Hangzhou, China) 1/16/30
Zhengzhou University (Zhengzhou, China) 2/14
Ziauddin University Hospital (Karachi, Pakistan) 15

ABOUT THE AUTHOR

Dr. Mark Fritz, NMD, PhD is President and Founder of *New Medical Frontiers, Inc.,* a leading international center for documentation and information about latest scientific breakthroughs in natural medicine.

Dr. Fritz has a career as an internationally renowned researcher in the field of holistic ecology and natural medicine.

He now focuses on information and education in, inter alia, Natural Cancer Support, Chronic Illness, Personalized Health Planning, and Second Medical Opinion, etc. - with special reference to research and scientific validation of renowned U.S. and international medical schools and research institutions. He also gives seminars on natural medicine.

His Academic Career includes:
- Researcher, Max Planck Institute, Munich, Germany
- Research Scientist with the United Nations in Paris
- Visiting Professor, Oklahoma State University
- Adj. Associate Professor & Associate Director of Natural Resources, University of Georgia
- Trainee in the Mexican Rainforest

His Board Certifications are:
- American Alternative Medical Association
- American Association of Drugless Practitioners
- American College of Wellness
- Federation of Independent Experts for Natural Medicine in the European Union
- European Economic Chamber of Trade, Commerce and Industry

>>><<<

Dr. Fritz is also the author of the medical books

MANAGE CANCER TREATMENT SIDE EFFECTS NATURALLY
(ISBN: 978-0692-58589-4)
&
BOOKS OF NATURAL HEALTH Volumes 1/2/3/4
(ISBNs: 9781797049977/9798626536287/9798402906082/20449798375574011)

For questions and/or interest in his books & seminars see website
www.newmedicalfrontiers.com
or contact: Dr.Mark.Fritz@newmedicalfrontiers.com

www.ingramcontent.com/pod-product-compliance
Lightning Source LLC
Chambersburg PA
CBHW050910260726
48660CB00001B/125